GRAY HAIR
ADVENTURE

Things I Learned About Life When I
Stopped Dyeing My Hair

SUSAN PAGET

SUSAN PAGET

YOUR FREE GIFT

Hey! I appreciate you buying and reading my book and as a way of saying "gracias" I've got a free gift that is exclusive to followers of my work.

I've created a Wellness Journal that lets you get on top of your spiritual, emotional, physical and mental health for 30 days. That means that for one whole month you're gonna get very clear on things like how you spend your time, how you really treat your body, the quality of people you hang with and the practices you use to stay sane.

Way too many of us don't pay true attention to our daily life. We just get through the day, but then we wonder why we don't feel right and end up at the doctor with our hands up in the air.

In this free workbook, I show you how to get conscious of your life and have fun doing it. I also love that this journal contains supportive daily affirmations that will help turn a month of investigation into a fun journey. To grab your copy, check out this link: http://www.thechangeguru.net

CONTENTS

INTRODUCTION

When I was 51 years old, I stopped dyeing my dark, blondish hair (well, in my *mind* it was blondish, but really it was orange!) and ventured into the weird, taboo world of letting it be its natural gray. Or at least I assumed it would sprout out gray. Honestly, I had no idea what exactly "natural" would look like for me, but it didn't matter. A switch had been flipped. Something in me said "Just do it and do it now." I was ready to take a chance, see it through and find out.

Not long after my last dance with frying my hair in foils, I started making monthly YouTube videos about the adventure as it happened. The timing was perfect. I'd just started a business focusing on writing, speaking and coaching women over 40 and not only was the subject right on track with my work, doing the actual nuts and bolts of scripting, filming and editing inspired me. I used to be a television producer and documenting the mystery that would soon be coming out of my head was a throwback to the creativity that I loved about my old job before I walked away from it.

My YouTube channel is a mere blip on the radar of channels out there and while I only have a small community now, before I did my gray hair videos, I had no community! I think I had about three subscribers and I'm pretty sure that was made up of my sister (Thanks, Shells!), a YouTube "bot" and some guy from Kazakhstan who I eventually had to block. So the bottom line was that I might not have had anyone watching what I did but I really had nothing to lose by putting these kind of videos up that exposed a vulnerable part of myself. Being entertained and expressing myself was enough of a reason to do it. So even though this is just the introduction and not even the real part of the book, I can't help but give you an important tip before we get stuck in and that is:

"If you have a creative calling - even if it makes no sense at all and no one will see it - answer the call. Now."

The reason why you really should just put that "thing" out there is because when your soul wants to create something, uniquely you, that calling <u>never</u> goes away. It keeps on nagging at you. It taunts like a mean girl. Of course, most people get used to not listening to this deep part of themselves and understandably so. It means we have to go outside our comfortable and safe square, but the deeper the longing, the better chance that it's gonna getcha, one way or another. Perhaps the light-bulb moment that says you should've gotten your creativity on comes in a crisis. Maybe it's courtesy of a life altering situation or the end of the road all together when we get hit with the big question of "Why didn't I do *that thing*? What was I so afraid of?" Listening and following through on one of these creative urges, even if it's just taking the smallest action is insurance against the boring and inevitable "I should'ves..."

So my creative calling was to document my gray hair and without too much effort, every month, I'd express it. Forget fancy equipment like cameras, lights or tripods. In the kitchen of my beachside apartment, I'd prop my iPhone against our latte milk frother thingy that I stuck on top of a cardboard box that my juicer came in and I'd talk about where I was at on the gray hair regrowth grid.

Along the way, I also journaled and a good chunk of these private thoughts are what make up the bones of this book. A warning. Some of the things that I share here are a little on the cringeworthy side but I learned pretty early in the gray game that there was more to this whole thing than the hair. Going against the grain and ditching dye was symbolic for a lot of the lessons that I happened to be knee deep in. Just about every problem that women I work with encounter, I had either tackled on some level, successfully or somehow navigated around it or was going through all of it in real time. The "going through in real time" is a tough one for me because I like to be able to give definitive answers. I like to share pathways that work. But this one, this gray hair thing, well I had no idea how it was gonna pan out. At the start I felt like I could complete the mission but what if I bailed half way through. What if it turned out terribly and I looked awful?

This concept, of not knowing what's ahead is so symbolic for the whole midlife and beyond experience. Other than an occasional celebrity, we've got very few successful references about how to not only get through the challenges of growing up after 40 but enjoy the journey. For now, most of us who want more are in the position where we've gotta white knuckle it.

So, if you're going through something where you feel like you're the only freak in the room, welcome! I hope that by me being transparent about this time, you'll feel less alone and spurred on to keep going even if you have no idea the direction you're traveling. Seriously, if I can do anything that I'm doing right now, you can too.

Here's something you may or may not know about my gray hair videos. Most that I made were done when I was feeling especially on my own. I was in the trenches of a total career transition, a midlife chapter that so many of us will consider, actually go through or avoid all together because it can be so tough. During some pretty challenging times, it felt wonderful to think about gray hair, what it meant beyond my head and how I could parlay that into a lesson about life and maybe help one person who was struggling. Man, I can't help myself but I have to give you another tip:

"When life is sucking balls, you must help someone - it will suck less."

You're welcome.

So the long story short is that this first year of my gray hair experience collided with a time where I felt very vulnerable with my new career direction. I loved it, but it was tough. It was lonely. It was exhausting. Many times it still is all of those. The saving grace for me has been that I know my purpose and that's to help people through communication and doing it in my own unique way. Gray hair gave me a kind of license to stay on track with this purpose even when I was on shaky ground.

This is where YOU come in.

Your prickly thing, the thing that is challenging for you right now can actually be supported by going on your own gray hair adventure. Let's say beauty, self worth and esteem are where you're feeling weak. We can work with that. Or maybe it's relationships or health. Going through this adventure, even if it's vicariously through me, might give you some light bulb moments.

Maybe you're surrounded by people who always tell you what to do or you've got people in your life who think it's fine to cross your boundary lines of appropriate things to say. Fantastic. My story is for you. Whatever your "thing" is, if you're open to going deep, the gray hair adventure is an incredibly valuable journey for cleaning stuff up and dealing with these things once and for all.

As each strand of silver has sprung out of my scalp, I've learned lessons about life and those are the things I've put in this book. My big, huge hope is that whether or not you're ditching dye, you can use my adventure as a way to get really solid about your own, and I'm talking about the adventure *beyond* your hair.

P.S. A little housekeeping before I get started. After a couple years of videoing, talking and writing about gray hair, I'm still not clear whether you spell the word with an "A" or an "E". It seems that it depends what country you're from which is a challenge for me because I'm a dual American and Australian citizen and both countries spell the word differently. From the beginning I went with my American roots - get it, roots?!! - and stuck with grAy. And that inspires one more tip in this introduction:

"Don't be afraid of your roots"

QUEEN
OF
THE SILVER SISTERS

You know about Cindy, right?

If there's one woman who personifies the possibilities of what happens when you embrace your natural gray hair, I'd say, you go to the source. You'd have to go to the supermodel for the boomer generation, Cindy Joseph.

Now I have a feeling if you've picked up this book, you know who I'm talking about. If you don't, I need you to stop what you're doing right now and Google her. This is important for context. Otherwise you might completely miss the impact this woman has had on the concept of not having to dye your hair anymore. You need to see Cindy to believe what I'm saying because with one look, if you had any doubt, I reckon she will completely 180 your brain when it comes to what you thought you knew about older women and gray hair.

Cindy Joseph was a big part of my arsenal for making a slam dunk case to family and friends (not to mention myself!) that I wasn't out of my mind to stop dyeing my hair. I relied on Cindy as kind of a "one stop shop" for letting my inner circle know that what I wanted to do made sense on a lot of levels.

Like all awesome role models, there's some very cool lore attached to Cindy Joseph's role in the gray hair movement. Legend has it this way. Cindy was walking down some New York city street in her late 40's, her long hair had just had the last of its dyed bits cut out and her boyfriend had encouraged her to never color again.

Can we just stop there?

Cindy had a *boyfriend* who actually *encouraged* her to *stop* with the dyeing business so she could rock long silver hair.

Between having a boyfriend (because so many midlife single women stress out about never meeting someone) and being encouraged in a decision that so many women worry will turn men off, Cindy had me at Hello!

So, the story goes that the DAY she cut the dyed bits out of her hair and was walking down the New York street as a midlife woman with her silver glory flowing on down, she was spotted by a Dolce & Gabbana talent scout and signed on the spot.

A silver star was born.

From there, this natural beauty of a woman who wasn't afraid to embrace her age and the obvious signs that she was living it, caught those who were looking for a light at the end of the beauty age tunnel by storm. Super Cindy became a sort of poster child for what was possible if you dared to play the cards that nature and age dealt you.

And she did it on two levels. Even though I don't imagine Cindy to be the type to give the middle finger to anything, in my mind, in her own gracious, regal way she did just that. Not only did she not dye it but she wore it long too. Because that's a "thing" also right? Somewhere along the road, someone decided that long hair is a "no-no" after a certain age. I have no idea where that rule came from but I certainly wasn't buying it and it was awesome to see that I wasn't alone in my thinking.

Gray hair. Long hair. This double whammy of rebellion against a beauty status quo delivered by a woman who was drop dead gorgeous was just about more than I could bare when I first saw Cindy. She was a "dye-my-hair-for-the-rest-of-my-life" deal breaker. Clad in blue jeans and a tank top, Cindy was picture proof that you could look ageless forever *without* looking scared. The concept packed a punch with me because I was always looking for the social proof that how you want to age is a choice. You can choose to act, look and feel "old" or you can still be in the game of life.

And I just realized. I haven't even gotten to the hair part of Cindy's story yet.

Here's the thing about Cindy's hair. When we talk about silver hair and women, maybe we think about what we've seen in the media, perhaps Jamie Lee Curtis' pixie or Dame Helen Mirren's snow white blow out. But Cindy Joseph's hair was kind of from another world of silver. Where it was silver, it was the perfect shade, a kind of white hot. It was the stuff of a Calvin Klein perfume ad, like a crisp white shirt or sheets on the bed of an amazing hotel. But it wasn't just that. The silver somehow morphed into darker tones that took on a steel bluish hue. It was a stunning color palette that honestly, I've never even seen on a silver haired *male* model.

The business of its color out of the way, the quality of Cindy's hair was also extraordinary. Hanging long past her shoulders, it had the gentle waves of a Kardashian except for the fact that the look she had was completely counter to any high maintenance business.

About the time that I discovered Cindy Joseph, she'd launched BOOM, a make up and skin care line she created for women of any age. In her YouTube videos, where she recorded chats called "Saturdays With Cindy", she demonstrated, with a clean face how she used her make up. And true as day, this phenom of a woman just glided a little slick of a stick on her cheekbones, lips and forehead, and just like her brand was called, Boom, she was ready to go.

Seeing a beautiful, older woman who erred on simplicity, in jeans and only minimal make up was a revelation. For one thing, her face was completely appropriate and yet her skin was stunning. She wasn't overdone with fillers and Botox. She really had a look that showed what happens when you actually take care of yourself for a lifetime and not just in a way that is a surface thing. Cindy Joseph was what happens when you do the inner work. Honestly I really have no idea what the hell Cindy Joseph's life is really like but to me she resonated a feeling of being at peace with herself that so many of us ironically have to work so hard to fleetingly feel.

Encountering Cindy in those pre-dyeing days helped me on another level. She let me entertain the idea that me growing out my hair gray wasn't necessarily a first class ticket to "crazy-cat-lady- witchy-poo" land. This was important to me. Based on the odd gray hair that made it's way out of my head before I'd book in for my regular dye jobs, I was on track for some serious wire sproutage. I seemed to have wayward silver antennas poking out of my head that could only be tamed with color. So thinking about what would happen without that coverage was pretty scary to me. But Cindy Joseph gave my potentially Brillo pad

hair hope. Her silver locks were as smooth and divinely woven

as an angel's. For all I could imagine, the woman probably had

wings and a halo but did her best to hide them so she could

appear as normal and as accessible as possible.

Ms. Cindy Joseph was *that* ethereal to me.

If I sound a bit obsessed about Cindy Joseph, you are correct. I

can safely say that it was Cindy that completely pushed me over

the edge when it came to me working out whether I should

plunge into the world of dyeing or no longer dyeing my hair.

I have to tell you, this is not how I usually operate. Sure I might

be interested in a fashion trend but to be so influenced by a

celebrity to do something that is so taboo for women is

something that I just don't do.

But the image of Cindy Joseph was kind of like a talisman of

hope as well as a key bit of the arsenal that I planned to use in

convincing my inner circle that this was something that I was

going to do.

And here's the main thing that stuck with me when I think

about my first knowing about Cindy Joseph - Queen of the

Silver Hair.

Cindy didn't look frightened.

I never realized how scared women are of getting older until I

started to think about not dyeing my hair anymore. Once that

veil was dropped, I saw that the fear was so strong. And

because of that fear, so many of the natural parts of ourselves

are becoming neutralized, frozen in time. The perfect example

of this is our foreheads. As I write this I know full well that I'm

probably the last of a generation that thinks it's okay to have forehead wrinkles. Look around to see what I mean, less and less women have them. There's still time for me to jump to the other side and maybe I will one day. Maybe having these lines will be as socially unacceptable as not keeping your nails trimmed or getting your teeth cleaned. I suppose the thing that stops me for the moment is that it seems like either way you can't win. It doesn't seem like the fear goes away along with the wrinkles.

But Cindy Joseph didn't have that look of being terrified of life. Before my Cindy discovery, I knew that, health and destiny providing, my mind could hold up and see me through to the end of time. But when it came to *not* doing Botox, to *not* injecting my face with fillers, to *not* coloring my hair anymore, what would happen? Would the world, my world really accept me? I felt in my gut that it would but I really didn't know for sure - until Cindy came along because she had *that* hair.

That beautiful long, silver, Rapunzel hair stood for a woman who was proud of herself, who was an ageless goddess. It was like she was practically offering up her hand to younger generations like me (okay not, that much younger, but for the sake of being dramatic, you know what I mean) and saying, "Don't be afraid. If you want to follow the old way of living, a life lived in fear, and dye your hair, go right ahead. But if you're ready to be yourself, then here, take my hand. Let me lead you into another world."

And so I reached out with my bony fingers and grabbed the angelic, lightly tanned arm of Cindy as she reached through a Pinterest picture. *That one where she's wearing a white t-shirt and looking like she's practically 16 even though she is more likely 5 or 6 decades older.* I took her and dragged her onto my iPad. On that day the device became my digital vision board for the proof that having gray hair was going to be okay.

Lesson Learned

Success leaves clues. When you need direction, find a role model.

When it came to my gray hair adventure, I lucked out because I literally had a MODEL as my role model. Score! That was great for a physical goal like growing hair out gray but you can use this approach for any intent. Find someone who stands for your values and emulates an aspect of life that resonates with you. Having this gives you some kind of direction and pathway to follow. It's a little bit like Hansel and Gretel leaving breadcrumbs. A good role model leaves clues from their life, their attitude, their way of moving through the world, that can get you "home." They don't even have to be someone you've met. If I would've waited for a woman with silver hair that I connected with, to show up and deliver her wisdom to me, I wouldn't be writing this book right now. Actually, I'd probably be sitting in a salon *at this very moment* with a plastic smock over my clothes and my hair wrapped in tinfoil. Finding the person who's doing the thing that you dare to do is probably only a search engine away.

ZE SHEEET HEETS ZE FAN

*"*You *weeel* look like *sheeeet"*

I was sitting in the chair of my local salon. It's a place with a pretentious name, French staff, overpriced services, minimalist decor and a hairdresser who was totally losing *eeet.*

Most of the time, the salon was deserted, without a customer in sight. I always wondered, with so few clients, how they could possibly pay the rent even with services at a premium? And why was I there? It definitely wasn't my style and under normal circumstances I wouldn't have even stepped foot inside but the sad fact was that I had pretty much burned my way through just about every salon in my little beachside suburb of Sydney, Australia.

No exaggeration. *Okay maybe a little exaggeration.* It seemed like I'd been everywhere! And this was kind of a drag because in a small town like mine, I had no choice but to confront my past.

Every time I went in to do errands, I also had to do a walk of shame past these salons gone bad or more embarrassing, I'd have to run into the colorists I'd never rebooked with again in the supermarket check out lines. #awkward

The pattern of breaking up with hairdressers went something like this. Sometimes we'd have a decent run. I'd book in for an appointment *or three* but inevitably there'd be a problem and it would be over. Doneski. And of course, the problem was always about color. Always!

The situation would go down like this. I'd go in for "regrowth," hairdresser speak for covering gray roots with some blonde highlights added for interest. When the moon was in the seventh house and Jupiter aligned with Mars, the colorist would totally crush it and I'd walk out of the salon feeling like a million bucks. This was always a one-off.

With each second appointment, I learned that the hair color I walked out with was more about luck of the draw than any specific technique. Sho'nuff, the next visit would range from mediocre to downright horrible and in need of a fix somewhere else.

In defense of hairdressers, I totally get that coloring hair is much like a science. In fact, whenever I'd talk to my various colorists and ask them how they concocted their potions, my eyes would start glazing over. I'd give up thinking and just let them do their job. Perhaps I should've made myself learn the exact formula for the color I wanted? I don't know how far I should've taken it! Instead I treated the hair color game like basic gambling, with fingers (and toes) crossed.

I have one more "in defense of hairdressers" I want to add. My hair is no picnic to work with, especially as years of dye began to take their toll. I was told that my hair was "porous" and

"coarse" and "damaged". I was told it "threw red tones" and
that the "cool" color palette I always hoped for was impossible.

But this time, in the Salon *Who's Name I'm Still Not Sure How To
Pronounce*, things were gonna be different. I could feel it! And
more than that I was prepared. I'd been sitting with the idea
about jumping away from dyeing my hair for a couple months.
My iPad had become a virtual vision board of gray hair
goddesses like Cindy so I had a strong visual. I even joined an
online community called Cafe Gray, a private Internet group
where women posted pictures of themselves in dye free
transition, discussing in depth the process of growing their hair
out and sharing tips on how they put up with the Mother of all
Ditching Hair Dye Concerns - the line of demarcation - the
contrast between the outgrowing gray and the dye that used to
cover it up.

Whoa. Wait one minute. Transition? Line of demarcation?

What? It might seem obvious but I really didn't think this one

through. I mean, what would it be like to be walking around

with two-toned hair in various stages of growth? How long

would it take? I had no idea what this would be like for anyone,

let alone me. But this was one of the many ways that Cafe Gray

was awesome. Besides being a living, breathing "how to" the

community was a real posse, helping anyone who wanted to go

on the gray hair adventure get through the vulnerable bits.

One of my favorite parts of Cafe Gray was also one of the

things that gave me courage to take on the unknowns like

transition. For their avatars, members would post pictures of

their different stages, showing off lines of demarcation between

hair that had been dyed for years and the new, contrasting

natural hair. In a lot of ways, it was like comparing battle scars.

And these weren't glossy, filtered pictures. Some women

showed themselves in the thick of it, describing their look like that of a "sick cat" or a "skunk" and asking for advice on how to cope when they felt insecure about what they were doing. The response was always wonderful. I know we often ask ourselves if we women are our own worst enemies, but Cafe Gray was proof of what happens when women choose to really support each other. It's powerful. The members were honest, warm, and an accepting band of women who were there to see members through from the uncertain start of their gray hair adventure well to the end. As part of my education, I read every post whether it was about what kind of product to use to how to get through bad hair days. Being on that site made me actually excited to be taking on this new chapter in my life.

But of course, this new chapter wasn't just about me. I might've been solid with the concept of it all but what about my husband Dale? Would this turn him off? We'd been married for almost three decades and the last thing I wanted was to give him the idea that I was letting myself go. It's a weird thing for me to even write, because Dale never gave me any reasons to feel insecure with my looks, but perhaps old conditioning dies hard. When you're young and falling in love, the idea of growing old together is a romantic and charming part of the equation, but here I was doing something that could be the actualization of that.

And then there were my adult kids. They're my best friends and I especially wanted my daughters seal of approval. If I could get this thing right, then they'd have an in-house reference to back their own unusual decisions now and down the road.

So when the time came to see what my family thought, I turned on the iPad to all things Cindy, passed it around and said:

"Guess what guys? I'm gonna grow my hair out gray!"

And they were immediately on board. I think my girls even

broke out with a "Yay!"

That's really all it took. It was a no-brainer because I was

confident and there was no arguing with what they saw on the

iPad. It was a big hurdle to cross and while I still had no idea of

what was to come, I figured that every reaction I'd get would be

the same.

Wrong.

The hairdresser was a young French guy (the salon really was

into the whole French thing!) and honestly, I thought he got

me. In past visits we had semi bonded with our mutual love of

our local beach. He and my family were all surfers. We'd talk

about fashion, music, lifestyle stuff; the kind of generic talk that

goes on in the chair. And besides everything, he was French! He

had the blood of a country that epitomizes beauty and style and effortless chic running through his veins. I thought that of all people this hairdresser, who had to be on top of trends would congratulate me and actually be excited to take on the challenge of helping me through it.

But instead, I watched the color momentarily drain from his face before his cheeks and neck turned the color of a hearty Bordeaux.

He immediately lost his shit and I was completely stunned. In fact, I really can't recall anytime in my life when anyone was so vehemently opposed to something that I physically wanted to do. No one ever challenged the way I dressed or got angry at me because I didn't wear much make up. No one ever had a word with me because I didn't have breast implants to "improve" my silhouette after breastfeeding three kids. I always seemed to be comfortable in my skin. While looking cool was important to me, feeling comfortable was part of that and I thought that translated to people who knew me as well as strangers.

"You can NOT do *theez*," he sputtered. "Eeet can not be done, eeet eez going to look so *terreeble* and what's going to happen eez that you are going to try *eet* for a few months, and *zen* you're going to see how *terreeble eet eez* and *zen* you're going to come in here CRYING because you have done *somesing stupeed* and have tried to *feex eet* yourself and *zen* I will have to try to fix *eet* and *eet* will be complete *sheet*."

You might like to know that while he was yelling at me, he was looking at himself in the mirror. I know this is a hairdresser thing but I remember thinking as sort of a sidebar that he was actually checking himself out, anger and all, while he was slamming me. #impressive

You might also like to know that he had me checkmated. I could barely speak.

"But... I...I," I stammered, my face also starting to match his shade of Rose'.

And let me tell you something. it was such a weird dynamic. Here I was, old enough to be this guy's mother, not to mention THE CUSTOMER, but as a hairdresser, he had me by the short and curlies with some strange magical hairdressing power.

It was only after the fact that I realized just how much of an authoritative strangle hold these hairdressers in my life have had over me. I'm usually pretty good with directing people. It's a skill I've always needed for work as well as other areas in my life. But having clear communication with hairdressers was obviously lost on me.

Maybe you can relate. On one hand, I figured that for the money I was paying, a hairdresser would *have* to know what would work for me and on the other, I assumed that this was their career. They were in the business of making me feel and look as beautiful as I could be. And besides that, they worked with thousands of women, certainly they'd seen *everything*. I really put my hairdressers into the same authoritative box as I did my doctors and dentists.

This realization was a first for me. I thought of all the authority figures in our lives and how the notion that they were beyond reproach was completely ridiculous. Actually, it was beyond that. Not asking questions or pointing out wrongs was childish and potentially dangerous. This was absolutely one of the earliest big picture lessons that I got from going gray.

Meanwhile back at the hairdressers....While he continued his spray of outrage at me, I remembered that I hadn't even brought out the big guns. My iPad was still sitting in my purse when something inside me whispered, "Cindy, I need you!"

"Wait a minute," I tried to smile calmly, accessing as much mental aikido as I could muster to blend with his energy rather than combat it. Pulling out the iPad I muttered as matter-of-factly as I could, "Let me show you these pictures so you can see what I'm talking about."

Talk about a waste of time.

I don't think 10 seconds had passed before he completely brushed it off. He wouldn't even look at it until I specifically enlarged the picture of Cindy that had instantly gotten my family over the line, practically shoving the iPad in his face.

"Photoshop!" he snorted, adding "There *eez* no way that silver hair looks like *thees*. *Eet* eez lights, Photoshop, false!

And with that, I was done. I had pretty much shut down, losing any will to keep up the fight mainly because I knew there was no point. I did know one thing. It would be the last time that I'd be going to this hairdresser. The irony wasn't lost on me that in firing this dude, I had officially dug a hole for myself. I was a gal going through this gray hair thing without a local beauty salon in my corner to help me get through it. Funny the things that go through your mind when your hairdresser is completely hating on you.

The appointment was just for a trim so there was no further arguing about hair color. But it was one of the most uncomfortable cuts I've ever had. I could feel the venom of his feelings about what I was going to do through the shampoo. During the trim he seemed to cut more off than I asked for and I didn't say anything about it. When he blew it dry, the hot air seemed to burn the tips of my ears and the pull of my hair against the dryer to straighten it seemed forceful. Maybe it was all on purpose, maybe it was all in my mind and I was just ultra sensitive in defeat.

Through the reflection in the mirror, I noticed the only other client in the cavernous salon, a small woman who had to be well into her late 70's, maybe her early 80's. Her hair was being dyed a harsh black. There was no love or kindness being given to her as a cherished elder who was willing to pay big and still wanted to look good. I wondered if she heard the argument that we'd been having. She didn't look at me.

When the hairdresser finished the blow-dry, I'm sure he knew this would be the last time that I'd be making an appointment. And during those last blasts of hot air, I have to admit that I wondered if maybe I *was* crazy to think this was a good thing. Maybe over in the US, the movement of going gray had some kind of traction, but I was in Sydney, Australia. This was the land of a lot of blondes and that sunny, quintessential Aussie look was alive and well in this town.

I looked out the floor to ceiling glass windows and onto the streets outside and certainly didn't see any Cindy Joseph types walking around. In fact, the only place I'd really seen this type of vision was online. Up until this point I was so confident in what I was doing but now, I felt like I'd maybe made a decision based on a fantasy and one that was going to make me look, and feel, like *sheeet*.

Lesson Learned

Question everything and everybody.

Most of us have grown up to have a healthy respect for

authority and that's a good thing. But the key word is healthy.

At midlife I started to really see how so called "authority"

figures didn't always have my best interests at heart or maybe

even didn't have the same knowledge that I had. I've

experienced this with "expert" doctors who aren't up with the

latest information and don't integrate a mind/body/spirit

approach to health. Bizarre but common!

Putting our well being and decision making into the hands of

others, just because they fit the authority role is unfair not only

to ourselves, but to them. No one person should have to

shoulder the full responsibility of another. That means we have to come to our relationships with "authority figures" whether it's our doctor or our hairdressers, from a new lens. I'm now looking to these people who can help me with my well-being as partners and sometimes even employees in the business of "me" rather than giving them the power that practically turns them into my boss.

WHO'S AFRAID OF THE BIG BAD GRAY?

I'm not sure how it happened but being afraid of looking older was something that never entered my consciousness. That was UNTIL I stopped dyeing my hair.

I know, I know! What took me so long?

Even though I was right in the bulls-eye of the target demographic of women who are constantly being reminded that youth rules and to be petrified about that and to buy the latest goop to counter it, being afraid of my looks as I got older was something I somehow managed to ignore.

I'm not saying that I've never had issues with my looks through my life. Puhleasssse. Battling against my face, body and hair has been an overarching theme for like, forever. I just thought that's normal and what we humans do. I didn't see lack of looks as something that happened when you entered a certain age category because it was a constant from the time I discovered mirrors were important, like when I was a pre-teen and got my first horrible zit. I can still remember it to this day, a big, honking thing in the crease of my nose. It was practically a second nose. My mom showed me how to squeeze it and with that, it was "game on" with feeling insecure about my looks.

My skin was bad through my teenage years. I could never get a handle on my acne. I tried every drugstore product on the shelves in the 1970's - Clearasil, Sea Breeze antiseptic lotion, Buf-Puf scrub pads. I even went on antibiotics of some sort (those worked but I never followed up for future prescriptions), but you name it I tried it, including lots of baking my face in the sun to burn the zits off, a move that I'm paying for with just as much sun damage right now. I remember at the time there'd be warnings about what the sun would do to our skin when we were older. It made no difference at all. I couldn't even fathom the idea of being older and didn't think twice when I covered

myself with Vaseline or baby oil. #burnbabyburn

My skin issues clashed with a time where I became very self

conscious with my weight to the point of having a nice flirtation

with anorexia. I didn't even get at the time that I had a disorder

worth mentioning because it was kind of what you "did" in my

San Diego high school circles. We starved ourselves on diets of

a few hundred calories a day and were damn proud of it. We

then got some reinforcement of our extremely good self control

on the scale and then binged like there was no tomorrow.

I never got so skinny that my parents had to do an intervention

and I never had the guts to stick my finger down my throat, but

let's be clear, I was definitely a product of trying to live out

some kind of twisted idea of control and perfection. Fear of not

being loved because of how I looked was a very real constant

during my younger years. In fact, I really don't remember much about going to school but I sure remember doing math of the day's calorie-spend in my head.

Things changed for me when I met Dale. I met him at my heaviest. My punishing diets and excessive workouts were backfiring on me and I was just getting fatter and fatter. Funny that.

But he liked me, for me. This really was nothing short of a miracle.

Dale was from Australia and in those days before life became so connected and globally same-same, there was a really big difference in cultural attitudes towards food between these two countries. When we moved to Australia, I noticed that women were much more at home in their bodies than my California peers and that people didn't seem so obsessed with what they ate to the point of restriction or latest fads. Portion sizes Down Under were normal. It seemed like people loved being outside and being active, not for the sake of burning calories but because it was fun. #whataconcept

This was the early 80's and I suppose now there really isn't a whole lot of difference between both of my countries or the world in general anymore. But in those days there really was an obvious difference and it gave me permission to give up this dumb fight against myself. I finally relaxed and let go of the painful things I was doing, all in the name of trying to fit an impossible mold. It didn't happen over night but it was steady enough so that it wasn't forced and became a part of me. With every pregnancy I went through, I learned to nourish myself and be appreciative of my body rather than abuse it. I enjoyed eating well and balanced. I no longer dieted or weighed myself. All those things got me to where I was finally "normal" and not obsessed.

Through the years my eating habits have been pretty much the same. I'm grateful for the abundance of food available to me and I know when to stop. I use food as energy and not as an emotional friend. I also don't see it as an enemy. Beyond eating, I learned how to practice yoga, one of the key tools that's taught me to be kinder to myself. I also use walking as my main form of exercise. For a lot of years, my walks were pretty hard core and I distance trained. At the time it felt right. It felt good to push myself.

Oh and get this, maybe my "teen on a rampage" hormones finally chilled out or there was something to be said for all this self contentment but my skin, which was once my worst nightmare, eventually cleared. That was something I had only dreamed of.

To get to this place was a process. But when I turned 50, that's when things really started to change.

I reached a very distinctive fork in the road of how I needed to treat myself as I was getting older and my body was changing. It probably came about because for the past couple years I'd been "head down bum up" studying women at midlife and soul searching about what I needed to do to feel good during my own transitional time. I was really tuned into the frequency of what my mind, body and soul were telling me and maybe it was the first time in my life that all of these elements came together.

It was as if inside me, there was a waving of a white flag. It was time to surrender the fight for good. My intuition literally said "I'm done!" The war with myself was officially over. Kaput! I knew right away that there'd be no more boot (or bootie) camps at this time in my life. I didn't want to push myself to the brink to prove my self worth or to lift my behind in a direction it was never going to go. And it was more than my body. For the first time in my life, I was ready to do more than just appreciate my finally calmer skin. I wanted to smooth oils on it and tell it

thank you. In fact, I wanted to tell every moving part *in me* and

on me - that I was just fine the way I was.

Something in my being came to a place where I just really

wanted to make peace with myself. Even with its lines, my face

reflected a calm, happy person - and that was even when I had

my glasses on!

And my body felt perfect for me. The years of looking after

myself with yoga and walking gave me a naturally healthy shape.

And besides that, I'd had good health all my adult life. I'd had

three children. It was incredible what a machine my body was,

even with every imperfection. I couldn't justify not being

appreciative about it.

The fact that wanting to smash the bathroom mirror wasn't a

regular thing for me was kind of a miracle given that so many women I know don't feel this way. I often try to excavate what

was it that gave me this sense of backing my physical self? I had

the same kind of hang ups and faced the same kind of media

pressure that women worldwide are constantly thrown but

something in me was just not willing to give in to the idea that

not looking like a supermodel meant I was a defective human. I

think what gave me the edge when it came to comfort in my

skin was my mother's attitude towards beauty when I was

growing up.

If there was, and is such a thing as the opposite of a narcissist,

my mother was that. She rarely wore make up, never got her

hair professionally done or seemed to read a beauty magazine.

As she got older, she'd occasionally bum out over a friend who

had their eyes done and would get really disgusted over the idea

of any kind of surgery or injectable. Now that I think about it,

the only time that I really remember my mom demonstrating

any kind of obvious beauty self care was when she'd spend a

few hours on a Saturday coloring her hair. She did it herself,

sometimes walking around the house wearing an old t shirt,

sweats and a towel draped around her shoulders, her hair

covered in the color.

On one hand, this was a healthy mom for a girl to have. For

one thing, I knew that any success in my life had to come from

my smarts. I didn't grow up expecting that I was going to get

any breaks based on how I looked. In this way my mom was a

wonderful barrier against any typical media messages that

wanted to tell me otherwise. And she had character to back up

her lack of concern for anything but the most basic

maintenance. She seemed to totally own her decision to not

follow the women and beauty herd.

As time went on though I realized that I valued beauty in a

different way than my mom did. I like to spend time caring for

myself. It makes me feel better. It helps me stand taller. It's a deservability thing for me and it's something that I hope has been passed on to my own kids. Feeling beautiful, feminine and confident in our own unique skin is a right. My mom is always naturally beautiful to me but how I wish she would've experienced more pleasures of being able to nurture and appreciate herself. The concept of appreciating ourselves is sort of a new thing really and perhaps my generation is the first to embrace the idea that it's okay for us to do so.

So when I think about what got me to this place, of having (what feels like) a healthy appreciation of my own version of beauty, while at the same time knowing my exterior is not the part that counts, I have to credit the positive aspects of my mom's influence on this part of my life.

Regardless of how it all evolved, the timing of being content and appreciative of my own version of beauty was super important. I learned to see the current moment as an essential set up for how I'd feel about myself 10, 20 and 30 years plus

down the track. At 50, I learned that If I could develop a self

respect and appreciation for where I was right at the moment,

then I would be forever protected from the concept that age

meant I was supposed to feel bad about the evidence of time.

But then I decided to stop dyeing my hair.

All of a sudden, funky jolts of fear about my looks, that I'd

somehow skipped over for most of my life, were well and truly

there. And they were all the typical fears: fear of not being

found attractive, fear of being rejected in the workplace, fear of

feeling invisible, fear of looking in the mirror and despite all my

great self talk, not liking what I saw.

I thought about what these fears meant to my world. I'd gotten

the thumbs up from my husband and kids but what would my

extended family and friends say? While I always thought I

"owned my age" I'd now have to step up and face where I was at on the timeline. This was a new world to me.

I'd been one of those people who often got complimented for looking younger than my real age. I have to admit, it was fun to be flattered like that. What gal doesn't like her ego stroked? But, um, let's get real, in the back of my mind I knew that's just the kind of stuff you say when an older woman tells you her age. And as for viability in the job market, I was heading out on my own, so I didn't have to interview for jobs, but what if my new "older" look turned business away? I especially loved being relatable to women who were only just entering the midlife world but if I looked old, would it be a turn off? I thought of a lot of "midlife" focused websites that I'd looked for help from before I became a coach and many seemed, well, let's put it nicely, I couldn't relate to them. They weren't even close to what I envisioned for my midlife experience.

All of a sudden, my belief that I wasn't high maintenance with my looks seemed to turn inside out. I realized that I actually *did* care and that maybe, just maybe, my caring was motivated by an unconscious level of fear. That surprised me. It was like I'd been carrying some fear sleeper cell that all of a sudden decided to activate.

That fear, stuck deep in my bones, made sense when I looked into it. It's a lesson in basic biology. At its most core, attractiveness is what drives us to reproduce. When women were running around in prehistoric times, those most likely to be dragged into the cave (wink, wink, nudge, nudge) were the ones who were oozing estrogen by way of thick hair and great boobs. Keeping a tribe growing meant safety in numbers, more people to contribute to a society and ultimately survival. To not be attractive could literally be a death sentence.

This basic explanation is pretty much embedded in our

psychology so our go-to reaction when our attractiveness is

challenged is fear of being excluded from our tribe. The modern

world's addressed this as our life span has extended by creating

ways to keep us "cave-draggable." Ensuring our hair sticks to a

certain color that subliminally keeps us thinking that we're

younger (and in turn won't be pushed off a cliff by the tribe)

was something we just did. No questions.

I think we all know that the Internet changed everything. For

one thing we were able to have a conversation with others and

at least ask questions like:

"Who said we *have* to do this?"

"Who says I won't look sexy if I have my hair its natural color?"

"Who says that gray hair will really make me look older?"

"Who says that I can't get a job if I don't dye my hair?"

All these "who says" types of questions were, up until maybe just a decade ago, untouchable and really unanswerable. But because of the online world, a conversation was started.

And then of course, once photos could be added and videos could be stuck up and Facebook groups could be joined, things started to change. With lifetimes of hiding from gray and embedded fears still simmering beneath the surface, I knew for myself that there was still a whole lot of untangling to do.

So this was my test I thought. It was my time to look at this embedded fear that sprung from all these "unknowns and what ifs." I had to brace myself for answers to questions like "Who says?" or "Would I still be attractive to my husband?" or "Would I look old before my time?" or "Would I be relatable to clients? And as my *ex*-French hairdresser predicted, "Would I end up really looking like *sheeet?*

Lesson Learned

The only way "out" is in. Feel the fear and face it.

It was really helpful in my early days of growing gray to work out where my fear about it came from, especially because that emotion hadn't been common for me in other areas of my beauty story. From there I learned that my fear was purely based on the unknown.

Something I mention a lot in my work is to just flat out ask yourself "Is this real?" "What's my proof that I should be scared of all these fears I'm creating in my head?" It really is so fascinating how we can get ourselves completely worked up into a fear lather, exaggerating every negative scenario without investigating the truth of the fear and where it's coming from. When I genuinely couldn't prove that I had anything to be afraid of, I just gave myself permission to feel the feelings but I reframed them to an adventure.

When you go on an adventure, you don't know how it's going to turn out, but that's the whole point. I channeled the adrenaline of fear into allowing myself to enjoy doing something that was uncertain, rather than stay safe and have regrets. And this is something that you can apply to any place in your life where fear pops up. Reframe it into an adventure. You'll still feel the adrenaline but changing the way you think about it lets you use that energy in a way that encourages you to keep on going, rather than become catatonic.

JOINING THE CLUB

So I'm walking out of the *Salon de We Hate Gray*, and I looked around. Talk about getting dropped down to earth. There were no Cindy Joseph types in this town. And come to think of it, maybe there never was. I couldn't even name the last time I'd seen a smart looking gray haired women in the center of Sydney, let alone this little beach suburb. Suddenly, the "evidence" on my iPad seemed kind of delusional. My hair might've been freshly blow dried which always calmed down its natural wildness, making me feel more polished, but the $189 (*omg!*) I'd just forked out was a big waste of cash, not to mention time, for how it left me feeling. I was shitting bricks inside and on the way home I see-sawed between being freaked out and totally infuriated.

As soon as I got home and through the front door, I made a bee-line for my laptop and Cafe Gray. Even in the short amount of time that I'd spent there, I knew that there'd be a kind member who'd be able to talk me off the ledge. It didn't even matter that I was on a time zone at the other end of the world, the community had an uncanny way of having someone on board 24/7.

There was a refreshing old school quality with the Cafe Gray message board that actually worked in its favor against the backdrop of so many Facebook, blogs and Pinterest pages springing up around the gray hair movement. That quality was privacy and a genuinely supportive group atmosphere with members who'd been there since the beginning rather than random visitors.

I wasn't surprised to discover that Cafe Gray was created by Diana Jewell, who in my mind is one of the first people who really connected the dots between going gray and beauty for *all* women, not just celebrities. For a few years before I'd taken the plunge myself I'd seen her book "Going Gray, Looking Great" and was pretty astounded by what she'd laid out. Diana was able to take the subject and show in full color, well groomed women owning their gray selves in a way that hadn't been done before. Cafe Gray was the same. It was a community that got in the game early and that turned this message board into the first port of call for women ditching dye. Even Cindy mentioned it in interviews.

Oh, the thought of being talked off the ledge by Cindy! #Idie.

The message board was made up of forums devoted to all stages of the transition, from deciding to do the deed to figuring out what type of make up would work best with it. The make up concept was an eye opener. It never occurred to me that the incoming color could totally change my palette. During these early stages I was more in "What the hell am I doing?" mode rather than "What color should my lipstick be?"

Other than my hair, color in general hadn't really factored into my personal style. I only did natural tones for whatever makeup I did wear and my wardrobe was full of black clothes. Chockers! It just made life easier. But now, here I was learning about options. This message board reminded me of my teenage years and discovering beauty products for the first time. There were tips and suggestions of what worked and what didn't and they didn't come from a magazine or a television show. It was secret women's business, a sisterhood at its best, supportive and honest but also proudly feminine. Going into Cafe Gray for the first time was kind of like in The Wizard of Oz when Dorothy opens the door in sepia to the Technicolor land of Oz on the other side. Speaking of Oz, that's Diana Jewell's nickname because of this new way she helped others look at gray.

I spent most of my time on the site as a lurker, preparing myself by looking at all the transitions and stages the members were going through. I had posted a few times when I was ready to take the plunge of no longer dyeing but now I needed to

workshop "the French hairdresser incident" and try to work out

what had just happened.

In my post, I relayed what went down in the chair, wrapping up

with the thought that even though I was pretty sure I was done

with him, I still had mixed feelings about cutting the cord for

good. I felt like a harsh decision would backfire on me. After all,

I'd burned close to all of my hairdresser bridges. While he was

no doubt out of line, I explained to the Cafe Gray gals that I

might be willing to suck it up and return regardless. After all he

was *pretty good* when it came to cutting my hair.

This was a pretty interesting example to me that even when we

think we're backing ourselves, if we're caught off guard, it can

be an all access pass for someone to cross our boundaries.

Looking back to this time, it's fascinating to me that despite all

the evidence, I wasn't 100% willing to cut this hairdresser loose.

Honestly, I should've known better. I was a coach after all and boundaries are a massive pillar of a practice but my defenses were down. I was operating in "little girl" mode.

This is where the women of Cafe Gray totally rocked. They weren't buying my flip flopping one bit. In fact, those women could sniff out bad hairdresser behavior a mile away and no sooner had I posted did they set me straight.

They pointed out that there was no way in hell I should go back to this hairdresser, regardless of what kind of way he had with a pair of scissors. His behavior was completely out of line. They also cottoned me on to the possibility that there was more at stake than any sort of customer care he had for my style welfare. It hadn't dawned on me that my decision to stop dyeing my hair was a matter of lost dollars for him. Was that really what the meltdown was all about? Maybe it *was* like a regular customer pulling the rug out of your business.

Whatever the reasoning behind it, the Cafe Gray posse talked me off the ledge and that's when things got good. My old journalist instincts started to come back to me and I could feel butterflies in my stomach. Whatever challenges I was going through, someone else had to be going through them too, right? And maybe they didn't know there was a Cafe Gray out there to support them. Maybe gray hair wasn't even their issue but there was something going on in their life that was parallel. Maybe what I was doing could have value and teaching and could actually do some good.

In my book *"How To Find Your Purpose After 40: The Secret To Unlocking Your Unique Gift To The World"* I explain something that hovers around spoiler alert material. If you haven't read it yet, skip ahead, or on second thought, never mind, read this anyway because it sometimes takes us many experiences to get the truth. Living your life purpose is all about helping people.

It's not some big grand thing that needs a lot of attention and spectacle. Living your purpose is simply the act of extending yourself, with whatever your unique thing is, and helping someone.

Because of those die-hard producer skills of mine, whenever women share their biggest challenges with me, I get very excited. I see a book. I see a YouTube channel. I see blogs. I see a business and a brand. I know that sounds insane because of course not everyone sees the media as a pathway they want to go down. But I think that we forget how valuable our personal stories are to others. And not only that, there will never be another person, like us, who can tell it.

Perhaps one of the things that keeps us from wanting to "do" something with our challenge is that we don't think we're enough. We don't have the qualifications to share with others or we don't have enough connections. I suppose I could've easily taken this route with the gray hair experience. I was no beauty blogger! I had no clue - and still really don't - on just about anything hair related. Who was I to talk about it?

It was weird and maybe a little bit scary. If I chronicled what I was going through, it was going to add more unknowns into the direction my life was taking with my business. I had no certainty on whether people wanted to watch me talk about this. Was it a good thing, or a bad thing? I really had no idea other than maybe, just maybe, sharing the experience might help someone. Or at the very least it might be entertaining.

So I set up my iPhone and sat on a bar stool in my small kitchen and I just talked. I told the story of the hairdresser experience and then I shared a few ideas. I decided to use the gray hair as a device to turn what I was experiencing into coaching lessons that veered in the areas of self-esteem and healthy attitudes towards getting older. I was pretty sure it wasn't a stretch.

I uploaded the video, tried to add some graphics with the built-in YouTube editor and called it a day. I didn't get the type of mammoth views that a lot of YouTubers enjoy on a regular basis but there was a noticeable difference between this first gray hair video and the ones that I'd done before. And there seemed to be more traction on Facebook and on Twitter than usual. I was also able to use it as a topic that week on a new podcast I'd started.

I noticed not long after that, subscribers were signing up, a few at a time, but in larger numbers than before. Even at its most miniscule, it was just a huge relief that finally I was being heard. After so many months of trying to connect with people, it was almost a miracle that something I was doing was working.

Lesson Learned

Your challenge can become your courage and your courage should be shared.

In the scheme of things, growing my hair out gray wasn't going to create world peace or feed the hungry. It was just a little bump on the road of life that tested my feelings about age, beauty, self worth and boundaries. But by going out of my comfort zone and sharing the experience, people responded. In facing my stuff, rather than pushing it away, I was able to find inspiration.

How we tackle our biggest challenges can potentially make a positive difference to not only our own lives, but to others. Whether it's a hiccup or a worst case scenario, finding ways to make our way through the muck is the stuff that purpose is made of and from a business sense they can even be monetized.

So many times, I meet incredible women who are going through extraordinary and tough experiences that if they shared their process rather than feel ashamed, they could have the most incredible work to give the world. My gray hair adventure is a micro example of that. I've used my videos, podcasts and blogs to share my story and connect with followers and go figure, now it's become a book. I could never imagine that this thing that made me want to shrink with embarrassment in the salon chair would turn into a subject that would help someone find me. I didn't think for a moment that going on a gray hair adventure could help my business.

Often for midlife women, when we're in an extremely stuck place or in the suckiest transition, we can't see a way out. There's a quote that I love that dares us to face this place and it goes "The only way out is in." By sharing the thing that you're going through, whether it's through an online environment like I do, or via chats over coffee, or hanging out on a message board, your challenge can also be gifted as your purpose, a

purpose that serves on a personal level and even in a business

that is uniquely you.

PRETTY HURTS

Probably one of the reasons that I was able to take the plunge of ditching dye in the first place was because I lean towards low maintenance. You get that by now, right? I've said it in one way or another about 349, 856 times so far. Pretty much everything beauty related that I do is relatively minimal. Truth be told, I could probably stand to ramp it up a bit and usually once a year, I go through a stage where I feel like I need to learn, once and for all, how to wear eye make up or that it's time to paint my nails the latest color. I buy the trendy $$$ products, give them a red hot go for about a week and then Dale will tell me that my mascara is on my face or my nails are chipping and that's enough. I'm done!

The no-frills thing is probably a combo of what was passed down from my mom and the attitude that I'm kind of fine as is. I think all these years of taking care of myself shows, or at the very least I feel it on the inside and it gives me the confidence that I don't have to cover myself in a lot of stuff. I have to admit the time factor for my current routine is pretty sweet. I

probably can get ready quicker than some guys. I just put on

sunblock and a little concealer for the usual suspects - under my

eyes, a zit (by the way, these days I get very excited when I get a

zit!) - and then I pop on some lip gloss. The same thing has

gone with my hair. Most of the time I air dry it with the most

effort going to an occasional flat iron over it when it's out of

control! I've never had a blow dryer, leaving *that* to the

professionals, although one day, a DIY blow-out is something I

wouldn't mind learning.

When it came to coloring back in the day, I was a late bloomer

only because it never occurred to me that it was something that

I needed to do. It was in keeping with my "If it ain't broke

don't fix it" beauty belief. For one thing, my hair seemed fine

with this low maintenance approach and that even went into

how I washed it. I used the cheapest shampoos and

conditioners, had no idea about product or that you could even go to a hairdresser to get it blow-dried. Looking back even I can't believe how out of the loop I was with hair care. Maybe it was a pre-Internet thing?

I only attempted to color my own hair a couple times during my early 20's and that was because I always had fantasies about being a classic, cool, blonde. "Fantasy" is the perfect description because this look, especially in my own hands, was only "in my dreams"! To give you a visual of what a nightmare this home color adventure turned out to be, picture Dale (we called him "ViDale Sassoon" during this experiment) pulling my hair by the strands through this rubber hair cover thingy so that we could then paint them with highlighter. It seemed straightforward in the instructions, but whoa! Talk about a botch job. That was the first time that I learned that a bad hair day could cause tears. Ha, Dale got that message too! Safe to say, I never got that epic blonde look but I sure rocked a horrible shade of orange that somehow leaked through the holes of the hair cover. The next day I was in a salon to fix it and I suppose that's when I also learned that coloring my hair was a job for professionals, not for me (or ViDale Sassoon!).

I eventually let go of the attempt to go platinum and started to come to terms with my natural hair color. To me it was an unexciting dark blonde, mousey brown concoction but it was also healthy, totally virgin (except for the experiments of which we will not speak), untouched and un-blow-dried hair. And it matched my life. We'd been married for five years, had a family and had moved back to the States. We lived in a yuppie - hippie enclave of Southern California so the low maintenance thing was on trend.

But there were times when my hair seemed a little too much Haight-Ashbury for even my tastes. The color was unsophisticated and boring. It needed something. I started to think outside my low maintenance square and wondered if I'd have better luck with some streaks of blonde rather than a headful of it.

A hair coloring seed had been planted.

We moved back to Australia when I was in my early 40's and around that time I took the plunge to brighten things up. I didn't have any gray at all and from what I can work out, that wasn't a family trait. Or one that anyone admitted to!

As I started to get busier in my old media career I entered the new world of regularly getting my hair colored. It's part of the package of being a busy working girl, right? At first it was pretty simple. A bit of "me" time. Just a touch and no big deal. But somewhere along the line, the "just a touch", "part of the package" highlights morphed into streaks reporting for duty. My hairdresser at the time told me that my grays were coming in. How much was going on up there, I had no idea! No one offered to show me and I sure didn't ask, even though I didn't see any obvious signs in the mirror. I don't remember feeling upset that I had a "sign of aging" or a frantic desire to keep them at bay. This transition was distinctly unemotional.

This new stage welcomed me into a new club of top secret girl stuff full of ritual and lingo. When I'd book appointments, all I had to say was the code word "regrowth" and I was in the door. It was like Fight Club! The only thing was I was a rookie in this club. I thought "regrowth" meant refreshing the color from before but for the hairdressers it meant "cover all traces of gray." Maybe I really had no idea or maybe I chose not to get clearer on what was happening on top of my head, either way I didn't have time to deal with it. For all I knew I could have just one stray gray or it was full blown outbreak going on up there. It didn't matter. I just needed good hair so that I could work and look okay.

When I think back to this busy time in my career life, which also coincided with being a mom of three teens, it's pretty interesting how much of it was spent in various salons trying to hold myself together. It wasn't just about having good hair color. Like any busy city, Sydney's lifestyle was a hungry beauty beast that needed to be constantly fed. I ran myself ragged to get in the door for my regular manis and pedis, facials, Brazilians, full leg and eyebrow waxes. That didn't even count for the clothes, shoes and products that I had to buy to maintain all this action. And remember, I consider myself pretty low maintenance! I think I would've exploded if I had to add spray tans, make up, Botox and daily blow dries to this schedule.

Regardless, taking this trip down memory lane right now is pretty confronting. I'm 100% for looking after ourselves and indulging in feminine rituals, but laid out in black and white, it's clear that I spent a lot of time trying to keep myself to some kind of standard that I made up as being very important in my head. Certainly no one was holding my feet to the fire forcing me to color and pluck and rip at my body parts.

And there's another thing that I can't help but acknowledge and that's the *dolla dolla* bills of it all. Honestly, the amount of money that I spent doing all this was something I certainly didn't want to pay attention to at the time and I really don't want to do the math on it now. Let's just say it probably added up to a round trip overseas plane ticket with some level of accommodation thrown in. Cha-ching! In a way, it's a lot like how women with children have to work out if their income can really justify day care. It's funny too. No one really tells us to ask if our income really can justify the amount of money that we spend on looking the part. We just do it.

And man, I was wiped out and utterly exhausted during this time. How wiped out? Well, I'm pretty sure I was able to take power naps during Brazilians. Honey, that's *tired!!* I know at the time that all these rituals made me feel good and that they had to be done but I can't help but wonder if I was caught up in some weird cultural merry go round that's not really questioned.

And that really leads me back to that big question of "What was I thinking?" when I started to have my hair colored to cover gray. I never questioned the practically religious devotion to scheduling appointments to do it. I didn't even ask "How gray am I?" I just knew that as soon as I would walk up to pay the $200 something dollars (most often for a color outcome that wasn't really that great) that the receptionist would have me booking in for my next appointment.

At first that window to book in again used to hover around the 11 or 12 week window and that seemed pretty reasonable. But somehow the goal posts shifted and the time shortened to around eight to 10 weeks depending on how well the color held up. There were even times when it could be as little as four weeks if the color had faded and I had something important to show up for that couldn't hold out any longer. The more I colored, the more it seemed like I was in some crazy video game where there was a battle against covering the gray and the lasting power of the color used to do it.

No surprise that my hair, *if it had an option*, was not happy about any of this. Not one bit.

After a salon visit, when I shampooed on my own, my freshly dyed hair would instantly revert to looking dull and fried. No matter what I did, no matter what product I bought that promised miracles, my hair could never match how it looked when I left the salon. Those hippie California days when I did nothing to it at all seemed from another time. I couldn't believe that this was the same hair that was so far from fussy that I could practically wash it with clothes detergent.

The year before I stopped dyeing my hair, the window of time

between appointments was probably somewhere around every

six weeks and let me tell you, my hair was pretty much shot to

hell. No amount of conditioner, fish oil vitamins or magical

thinking could undo the damage that I'd done to it. Truthfully,

shaving it all off completely would've made sense if it wasn't so

extreme. I pretty much did the next best thing and kept my hair

in a tight topknot most of the time. It's something that I do

even now while I continue to grow out the fantastic

"craptastic", a reminder of what I did to my hair, and keep it off

my face and out of my eye line.

But getting your hair colored is more than a surface experience.

It's hard for me to think about those salon visits without

recalling the smell of the dye. I'll bet you can imagine it in the

same way if I say the word "lemon" and your mouth starts

salivating. I'm not a sensitive person but that smell. Wow. It's pretty hardcore when you think about it.

Then there's the actual *sensation*. It didn't register until I stopped dyeing but I recall how most of the time that I had my hair colored, it actually hurt my scalp. Like a burning feeling. Not to the point of damage, clearly as I've heard stories of other women who are well and truly allergic to dye and have screamed in pain only to see scalding and bubbling skin under the dye. No, my stinging was more in line with the "Beauty hurts" ethos. Just like it *hurts* when you get a Brazilian or it *hurts* when you get your cuticles cut out during a mani or pedi or it *hurts* when you get extractions done during a facial, getting my roots covered was the kind of hurt that I just chalked up to another thing to "man up" and take if I wanted to have at least *one* day of good hair until the next appointment.

I had somehow subliminally adopted the "no pain, no gain"

logic but I really don't know how that was passed on. I can't

remember one conversation with any of my friends about any

sensitivity or pain from dye and I never read any article about it

or heard it mentioned in the media. Not one hairdresser ever

said, "Let me know if this gets uncomfortable". I never had to

sign a waiver saying "Warning, when we use bleach in hair color

it might make your scalp a bit tingly."

Sometimes that ammonia smell and the "ever so tingly"

sensation that came from whatever was being put on my head

and was probably not okay, would hang on til I finally washed it

out with my own shampoo. It didn't seem right, especially for

the amount of money I paid, to have a head that didn't feel

soothed or smell good when I walked out the door.

And then there was the staining. This one hurt my pride. When

I'd come home from a color, I'd have a stain around the

temples and on the top of my forehead from the color bleeding onto my skin. It was a tell-tale sign for my husband of what I'd been up to that afternoon. Which kind of defeated the purpose of creating an illusion that this color was all effortless and "natural". If Dale saw it, why didn't the colorists? How was it okay to let me walk out the door like that?

I finally learned that this was a thing for me and I'd have to always remind them to take precautions to avoid it. Didn't matter. At the basin, once the color was washed out of my hair, the scrubbing to get the stains out would begin. And just as predictable, there would always still be a bit of color residue lurking in the tell tale spots. When I'd get home, the first thing I'd do would be to mix a paste of toothpaste into the stain and rub it out, a fix I found on the Internet. There was also another fix and that was to take cigarette ash and rub it in the stain. I passed on that one but the toothpaste version, which kind of worked, had its drawbacks. Because the stain was so close to the hairline it was near impossible to not get a little of the paste into

my freshly dyed hair. The result would be that there'd be

strands that would be a little gluggy to the touch.

I wondered if this was normal. Did everyone, even those who

worked with the best hairdressers deal with all this craziness?

The smells, the burns, the stains?

But I never asked these questions and I certainly didn't ask the

most obvious. Like, "Ummm, exactly how gray was I anyhow

that I was willing to endure all this insanity"?

So much for being in a career which was really all about asking

questions and getting clear on the whole picture. It never

dawned on me to investigate exactly how gray that I was and

whether I really needed to be so obsessive with visits. It wasn't

until I began transitioning careers from working in the media to

focusing on issues that impacted women over 40 that I started to come out of my fog with what I was doing. I finally started to get curious and asked a hairdresser exactly how much gray I had. And, yep, it's one of the salons that I can't go to anymore. Matter of factly, she told me I was about 75% gray. I was slightly shocked because that seemed like a lot. Maybe I was in deeper than I realized. Maybe all those appointments to cover it made sense.

I learned though that this percentage varied depending on who I asked. In fact, when my *ex* French hairdresser was blasting me for my decision to ditch the dye, he mentioned that my natural hair color was really only 30% gray. And he assured me that because I had such a small amount, I was doomed to have a mousy salt and pepper result that would just look old and sad.

Up until I had crossed the line and actually stopped coloring it, I never felt afraid of my gray hair. Feeling fear about it wasn't on my radar. This dyeing ritual wasn't about any emotion. It was just a thing I had to do, like I'd been brainwashed. It didn't

matter how busy I was or how many other places I should've

been than sitting at the hairdresser getting my roots covered,

missing an appointment wasn't an option. It didn't enter my

mind to question what I was doing or whether there were

alternatives.

A lot's changed for me since those days. I look back and know I

was doing the best I could with what I knew at the time but I'm

glad that it's no longer who I am. Maybe it was a good thing

that my generally low maintenance approach to beauty went

commando to the other side so I wouldn't miss out.

I still have my beauty days and I love them, but they're more in

line with self care than playing a part. I don't do Brazilians or

get my legs waxed anymore. It was fun for a time but the

novelty didn't last. Good old fashioned razors seem to do the

job. Once in a very blue moon, I do my own nails, usually while

I'm watching a movie at home with Dale. Other than that I just

keep them trimmed. I get my eyebrows done but it's taking a

long time to get them back from many years of being over

plucked and threaded. I still get my facials, but most of the time

they're from a therapist who works out of her home. There's no

weird smells or waiting for rooms to be ready. As for my hair, I

know I should "never say never" but I have a good feeling that I

won't be repeating what I went through during my "busy,

working lady" stage again.

Lesson Learned

Self care isn't about hurting yourself.

It's easy to move through life doing things without looking too

closely at whether they really need to be done. But then

something happens. Whether it's hitting midlife or no longer dyeing your hair, the pattern gets interrupted and all of a sudden you can see that what seemed normal might not really work anymore.

Me, not asking any questions about my hair coloring experiences, was probably in some ways a learned behavior of wanting to be a part of a crowd and also believing in the passed on chestnut of "pretty hurts". I wanted to look the part at work without discovering options that might've been more aligned with my lifestyle. And I also just assumed that any pain, either to my scalp or to my wallet was just the price you have to pay to be attractive.

But if you're willing to wake up, the reality can be a game changer. Look at your life. What's not working? Where are you tolerating pain and doing nothing? Where do you find yourself throwing money so you can "be like everyone else"? What are you choosing to stay in the dark with and why?

When you find the answers to these questions, the next logical step is to try and work out your history. Where did you learn how to do these behaviors? Where did you learn it was okay to cope with them? What are the cost of these actions on an emotional, spiritual, physical and/or mental level? If you're too afraid to do the math, a reality check might be calling your name.

YOUR SIDE OF THE LINE

When the hairdresser warned me that letting my hair go gray was going to be a big mistake it rattled me but it didn't shut me down. I was more stunned really that what I wanted to do provoked such a response. But what would've happened if Dale and my kids hated the idea? Would I have listened? Would disapproval that close to home be enough to derail the plan?

Because of my videos, I started getting emails and comments from women who said that they really wanted to stop coloring their hair but the people closest to them, their partners, their mothers, sisters, children and best friends were dead set against it.

There were some gray hair-blockers that stood out. They include the women whose own mothers weren't having any part of their decision because THEY (the mothers who would've been upwards of 60 years old) didn't want to be discovered for dyeing their own hair. Really? #nicetrymom

Then there were women whose children were stressing out about what their friends would think if their mom was gray. Would their mom be mistaken for the grandma instead?

Even without support of their families, the women that wrote to me still wanted to do this thing but they also didn't want to make any waves. They felt pulled in opposite directions and it was messing with their minds.

This was one of those times where the gray hair adventure really paralleled the challenges that a lot of women deal with in many areas of life and that's boundaries.

You know boundaries, right? They're that invisible, dividing line that separates the appropriate from the "don't even go there!" When someone crosses that line, you know it! The thing is, a lot of us don't say a word when it happens.

The concept of boundaries really seems to come up for a lot of women at midlife and I think one of the reasons why now, and not earlier is partly because this age can be a bit of a stopping point. It's like getting to a rest stop on a main highway with the only toilet for the next two hours. At the very least you have to decide whether to pull off the road or you have no choice but to get off at that exit and take care of business.

This "rest stop" that hits on the midlife highway is generally caused by some kind of attention getter like a health, career or relationship breakdown where we're forced to assess how our life is or isn't working for us. If you look really close you might see patterns emerging. We get a picture of whether we were the ones who made choices in the past or whether we let others take the reigns for us. We see what kind of people we've attracted and whether they've supported or kept us small.

It takes two to do the boundary tango. When someone crosses the line, you always have a choice of how you'll respond. You can step up and call it out or you can do nothing, allowing yourself to be steam rolled. No response is often based on a twisted reward. Going along with whatever's being imposed on you, even if it's against your grain, can keep the peace. It might seem like it keeps you safe. It can keep you feeling like a good girl even though you're seething inside.

During my time growing out my hair gray, I only had a couple experiences, other than the ex-hairdresser time, that got close to pushing my side of the line, but the fortunate thing was that I was able to understand that the opinions were more about the other people than about what I was doing. My gray hair was just kind of a conversation piece.

One time was at the pub with some girl friends in their late 40's who happened to be very "girlie girls" and would never in a million years ditch the dye. They made it loud and clear that what I was doing wasn't for them but that's as far as it went. We laughed. it was light and nothing more than conversational. There was nothing that they said that made me feel bad about myself.

I have another friend who thinks this is a passing fad and that I'll be back in the chair once I get it through my system. That makes me laugh. And there's another friend who just can't wrap her head around why I'm doing this at all.

What helps me so much is the fact that when you're completely confident about something it will trump anyone else's doubt. This is a killer statement to make about any decision you have to make, whether it's your hair or in your business or personal life. If something is important to you and you know in your gut that it's right, someone else's two cents on it might make you question yourself for a moment (like the French hairdresser did) but they won't shake your resolve.

What I love about the gray hair adventure is that it's a good litmus test for how you do boundaries in general. If you get pushback in doing this thing that's important - even healthy - for you, where else are people calling the shots in your life?

Which comes back to the question. What *would* I have done if my family gave me the big thumbs down on ditching dye?

I think that the way my family operates is that we say what we need to say but we have an overall respect for each other's choices. As long as no one's gonna get hurt, it's kind of okay. Knowing that, I think that they'd be able to have their opinion without crossing my line. I'd take it on board and keep going. If their responses really made sense, I'd weigh them against my own thoughts and give a little time to see if that changed anything. But you'll remember I'd done my homework, I knew what I wanted, my confidence in my decision would exceed their doubt.

The best way to look at boundaries, especially with gray hair is to consider the "golden rule." It's an oldie but a goodie that sums up allowing people to express themselves the way you want to express yourself. Especially if you're getting pushback on wanting to stop coloring, this is the time to do some self inquiry and ask whether *you* expect the same people to express themselves in a certain way. Are you supportive of *their* personal choices that might be harmless, but uncomfortable for you? How opinionated are you? How often do you want others to base their decisions on what's right for you?

They're tough love questions but boundaries are a two-way street.

Speaking of opinions, we live in a time where opinions are everywhere. The voiceless have a voice. A lot of us get confused when we think about the difference between being honest and frank with someone and venturing into places that are really just none of our business. We do this in the spirit of wanting to help someone "for their own good" or because we think it's funny. Or we don't even think that we might be crossing the line because we're not really listening to what's important to the other person. Now is the time where we seem to just like the sound of our own voice. It's like an audio "selfie." It's possible that someone's opinion on your choice is nothing more than hot air that will drift away to nothingness.

I also think the tolerance for where the boundary line is can vary in cultures. I know from living in Australia that you have to be able to have "the piss" taken about yourself, even among strangers. I actually love this. It's a frankness with a wink in the eye and I can give it just as much as I can take it. 30 years over here will do that to you. I have one friend who for months would tell me that what I was doing was a bad idea and that he didn't like it one bit. But he was also saying it in that ribbing kind of a way and it was hilarious. By the way, the other day he told me that "Actually, it's a great idea and it's perfect for you." Again, I just laughed because who knows what he really thought and it didn't matter anyhow. This kind of piss taking probably wouldn't fly back in my birthplace of Southern California where women, especially, seem to get super sensitive when it comes to opinions on their looks.

Regardless of where you live or who's giving their opinions, how you respond can make all the difference. Let's begin with how to respond to our kids.

HOW TO RESPOND TO KIDS

I mentioned I received a message from a mother whose high

school daughter begged her *not* to be gray at her graduation

because she was afraid she'd look like her grandmother. This

comment really stood out because we're actually in the middle

of a phenomenon where women, smack in the middle of midlife

are raising younger kids, thanks to new advances in fertility

options and adoption, so they might not be able to *help* looking

older. In fact, they might be the *same* age as some grandparents.

Many of these women didn't bank on the idea that through

raising their children they'd also be going through menopause

and confronting the issues of attractiveness as they got older.

They knew they might be more tired, but the subtle experiences

of aging were just as swept under the carpet as they are for

women who weren't in that situation. Their kids thoughts,

which are probably just a passing meaningless audio selfie

98

moment, have the potential, of really kicking these moms when they're down.

Can you see yourself as a mom in this type of situation? What's the best way for you to get what you want? Here's a script that will help you explain what you're doing in a way that opens the door for discussion while holding your ground at the same time. And while you're at it, truck out the reinforcements. Have visuals of women you admire rocking gray so your kids know you intend to look hot, not old.

SCRIPT FOR KIDS WHO DON'T WANT YOU TO DITCH THE DYE:

"Honey, I'm doing something that I think is going to be really beautiful for me but it might take a while, while it grows out to get there. I'm gonna ask you to respect my decision and to please cheer me on because it can feel wobbly sometimes!"

Note to mom: This is a two-way street. As long as your kid isn't going to hurt anyone or themselves with their choice, you need to return the favor and not nag at them about their fashion choices. I'm saying this as a mom whose daughter just shaved her head yesterday. #word

HOW TO RESPOND TO PARTNERS

The same gist applies to your partner. It was really important to me that I let Dale know that this wasn't about me letting myself go. This was a style choice. I wanted to look better for him. But it was such an off the wall thing to talk about, I remember feeling kinda vulnerable with it all. Having those pictures with me made a huge difference.

SCRIPT FOR PARTNERS WHO DON'T WANT YOU TO DITCH THE DYE:

"Darling, I know we're not used to seeing beautiful, sexy women with gray hair, but here's the look I'm going after (show your pictures). It's gonna test me while it all grows out but trust me, I want to look great for you and I know you will love it and want me to feel great about myself too."

Note to you: Walk your talk. Ensure that you support your partner's healthy and harmless choices. Respect his or her personal style. And here's a fun one courtesy of a very clever gal on my Facebook page. She suggested telling your partner exactly how much cash you've been dropping on those appointments to cover the gray. In this case, money might very well do all the talking you need.

HOW TO RESPOND TO MOTHERS

Mothers, and even friends, who don't want us to ditch dye are interesting. I never realized it until I started doing it myself but letting your grays come through can be interpreted as something *about them* rather than you. Your giving up dye means that your real hair will show and in turn will reveal what's actually going on with *them*. As always, have the Silver Sister power pics handy.

SCRIPT FOR MOTHERS/FRIENDS WHO DON'T WANT YOU TO DITCH THE DYE:

Mom/Friend: Dyeing my hair isn't a good choice for me anymore. I've seen some amazing pictures of women who are letting their hair be its natural color and I want to give it a try. I know what I'm doing isn't for everyone and there might be times where it gets tough for me as I grow it out but I'd love it if you can watch what happens and have fun with me while I go through it.

Note: If your mother or friends still talk you out of doing this, it would be a great time to do an inventory to see other ways they have made important life decisions for you.

HOW TO RESPOND TO HAIRDRESSERS

Even though I just get my hair cut or blow dried now, I still feel like I have to ensure I do my best to keep my boundaries from being crossed in the salon. I don't want to be asked if I'd consider adding highlights or covering all together, so my tactic

is to take the offense. As soon as I sit in the char, I say the

following:

SCRIPT FOR HAIRDRESSERS SO THEY WON'T BUG YOU ABOUT COLORING:

I'm purposely not dyeing my hair because I want to be gray so

make me look hot and help me work it! (and smile when you

say the "hot" part!)

Boundaries are complicated. If ours are being crossed, we have

to ask ourselves the question "Why?" We also have to ask how

often we cross the boundaries of others. When you ditch the

dye, you can't help but discover how well you draw that line.

Lesson Learned

Confidence in your choices must exceed anyone else's doubt.

Are you a pushover? Do you overreact? Do people tend to have their way with you? Do you walk away from conversations wishing you would've responded differently or called someone on bad behavior? If so, consider it an education. Most of us have been brought up to be good little girls, a concept that tends to get reinforced through the years not only in relationships but in the workplace. Feeling stung by someone's comment about your grays or feeling like you have to hold back on doing it to live up to someone else's standards could be a metaphor for other areas in your life where you've let people cross your line.

The great thing about using gray hair to address boundaries is that although it can feel like a heavy and important subject when you're going through it, it's actually a safe place to explore more serious areas. Most of the time, people that criticize your decision to grow gray just need more information and understanding of why it's important to you. Learning how to respond in a way that's respectful to the other person yet stands your ground, is an awesome starter for learning how to respond in more weighted circumstances where a boundary line's been stomped over.

HOW TO NOT
LET YOURSELF GO

My monthly YouTube videos introduced me to the world of the beauty vlogger. I seriously had no idea about what this was but clearly I was missing out on a social happening. From hosts that were "pretty damn young to know so much about make up" to "pretty seasoned and still couldn't get enough of it," this was a domain with its own gurus, rituals and secret passwords.

The surprising thing about the beauty vlogger phenom is that to be one you don't have to be an expert. You don't even have to be a model. You don't even have to have the nicest speaking voice. You just have to know your way around a lipstick and be absolutely obsessed by products.

And I mean ObSeSsED!

The crème de la crème of vloggers are YouTube millionaires from the advertising zoomed at the huge audiences on their channel. They've got their own product lines and television shows. They've got fans that scream when they meet them in person. I'm pretty sure the average players make a good living as well. In fact, even the small fish seem to have the audience numbers to be successful with ad sales.

If you've never experienced beauty vloggers, here are a few things I learned that might explain what you're watching:

Haul: The Urban Dictionary describes a haul as "in short, a shopping spree." While hauls aren't limited to the beauty space, beauty vloggers of all ages and popularity levels totally crush it in the haul department. Really popular videos show the vlog host laying out their haul and describing it in extreme detail. Sometimes hauls are the contents of their purse. Other times, it's what they picked up from a particular store. The packaging, the labeling, how much it costs, how big it is, how cute it is, what it will be used for - these are just some of the areas covered in a haul for each item. Judging by viewer numbers, audiences love watching these and request hosts to do them.

Empties: We apparently love to see that products from all those hauls have actually been used. In these videos, vloggers show their empty bottles and tubes and talk about their experiences with the products and whether they'll buy again. As much as the world of beauty vloggers is foreign to me, I do get inspired by the philosophy of actually using all your products rather than wasting.

Unboxing: Like it says. In the videos, vloggers take you through the whole unwrapping experience of products. I honestly don't think packaging has ever been so appreciated.

This world, where all things surface beauty are worshipped to the Nth degree was to me entertaining, occasionally educational, bizarre, mind numbing and overwhelming all at the same time.

Coming from what I've learned from working with women over 40, I'm not sure if this emphasis on the outer beauty, buy-buy-buy mentality and blatant narcissism is really that good for us. Because this content relies so heavily on the physical, it can be *another factor* that sets women up for the same trap that we fell for as teenagers, that we can never look good enough.

All that said, enough with the beauty buzzkill business. I just want to let you know that if you want to make gray to be a beauty upgrade, it's totally doable without doing hauls or orgasming over unboxing packages. The empties stuff though, that's something that's a good one to practice.

And you heard it right. I do believe gray is a beauty upgrade. It's a power move, even if one of the midlife beauty vloggers I just watched described gray hair with a "gasp." Even if an article I just read from an over 50 beauty expert said women doing the gray thing shouldn't let it grow long.

Whatever!

These are perfect examples of not letting people I don't even know cross my boundaries.

And those examples are where most thoughts on what gray looks like go. They head to that place of a woman who's letting themselves go.

So let's talk about that.

When I think of "letting myself go" whether it's because I'm not going to color my hair anymore or imagining what would happen if I stopped doing the other maintenance rituals that go along with trying to feel and look good, my mind goes to a bad place. I picture myself wearing clothes that make me feel invisible, a body I'm disconnected to and skin that lacks energy.

Diving deeper into what it would feel like for me to have all this disconnect from my physical self, I imagine that emotionally, it wouldn't feel pretty either. The idea of it all seems lonely and sad.

The option of letting myself go in this way is disempowering. It isn't being kind to myself. I don't buy into the idea that anything that suggests getting older - whether it's going gray or getting softer in our bodies - means we don't deserve to feel beautiful and work with what we've got.

I approached beauty and going gray as an opportunity to stretch myself, comfortably. When I took it on, I committed to stepping up my skin and fitness routines. I opened my mind to trying new looks and styles that would challenge or at least contrast the "old" connotations of gray. It hasn't been a drastic adjustment, it's more of an evolution.

When I started, I'd heard that my color palette would change and that clothes and lipsticks that worked in the dyeing days might not do the job now. I liked the idea of that challenge because like I mentioned, I verged on Angelina Jolie territory when it came to my love of black clothes. I loved the thought of experimenting with some new colors and even put a ban on buying anymore black clothes, unless I got absolutely desperate. That's something I am still sticking to. I did buy a charcoal sweater the other day but hey, every little bit counts!

My skin tone actually surprised me as the gray's have come through. I was expecting it would look dull but actually the natural color of my hair is much more compatible with my skin tone than the dyed. I'd also heard that the hair that comes out is more wiry and coarse, and while that's true for some of the hair coming out, I can tame them with product or styling. Beyond the wires, my hair has surprised me in how soft it's grown out. That's new for me.

Oh, I do have a beauty tip to pass along. you'll see it mentioned on one of my gray hair vlogs, so perhaps this puts me into the hallowed "Beauty vlogger" category. Hardly! But trust me, this is a good one.

One of my subscribers asked if I had tried "co-poo-ing". I had no idea what it was and after a quick search saw it's a version of the "no-poo" method. All this poo business boils down to not using shampoo and the co-poo method is for women, with curly hair like me, to just use conditioner to "wash" it. Not only do you just use conditioner but you actually don't rinse all of it out. I think the theory is that we put leave-in conditioner on our hair anyway, so why wash this stuff out? To dry, you wrap your hair in a big t-shirt or microfiber towel, which I actually think has been great for my hair as well, it seems less harsh than a towel.

The main rules of the co-poo method are to *not* use products

that have sulfates or any kinds of "cones" – those are chemicals

that include the word "cone" such as silicone, etc. That

intrigued me because I'd heard somewhere on the interwebs

that silicone was a friend to gray hair wires and the only reliable

product ingredient for holding them down. But taking it out of

my hair care was actually a better move for the look and feel of

it.

At its best, this method forced me to get *more* real about

chemicals that are in our products. It's easier said than done

though. I like being educated but holy crap, you have to work

for it. Most ingredients are written so small that it's an

excruciating, time draining mission to be an informed

consumer. My hunch is that the ones with the hardest

ingredients to make out generally are the ones with the most

junk in them.

But go figure. Ditching shampoo works for me.

After years of trying every product on the market and sparing no expense, an inexpensive bottle of conditioner changed my life. At least for now, but I'm optimistic. I can finally wear my hair down most of the time. The "co-poo" method is perfect for it and I have a feeling that this method, because it's so heavily moisturizing, would've worked during my fried, dyed hair days. I wish I would've tried it then.

Putting my coaching hat back on, I think that if there was one secret beauty weapon that we should keep close, especially through the gray hair adventure, it would have to be compassion. This is the time where tenderness for yourself needs to be front and center. For me, practicing compassion means checking in and asking "What's a healthy choice for me? "What will make me feel good?" "What can I do right now to feel better?" Or in times if I find I'm being hard on myself I straight up ask "What can I say to myself right now to be more appreciative and more forgiving?" "Would I speak to my daughter like this?" I find I'm constantly guided by this compassion. It might not come in a pretty box and certainly takes time and effort to cultivate but it is abundant and free, if you want it.

Here are five key, "beyond skin deep" beauty principles that I live by. They keep me from feeling like I'm dropping into the "let myself go" zone, especially during this gray hair adventure. What I love about these is that they are practically effortless and absolutely ageless.

1. **I love, respect and have immense gratitude for my body.** I know for some women it's almost impossible to say this sentence let alone believe it. For me though, I'm constantly in awe of the human body. How it works, how it

serves us, how complex it is. Even now as I sit here and write, I think about what it's taking at this moment for my brain to transmit signals that convey my thoughts into sentences and then instructs my fingers to type them out. How could I not want to do something that keeps those muscles strong? How could I not want to do something nourishing for my brain - whether it's writing this book or learning something new or ensuring I put good fuel into it. I try my best, to be in a constant state of gratitude with my body, even when my pants are too tight or I'm feeling self conscious in a bathing suit. And you know what's really crazy? The more gratitude that I can feel for my body, even with every imperfection, the more beautiful I become to myself. I think it's because I'm seeing myself beyond the reflection in the mirror. I'm seeing the whole person. If you have any doubts about feeling gratitude for your imperfect self, I double dare you to say the affirmation "I love, respect and have immense gratitude for my body," every day, every time you look in the mirror. This is actually a practice that I learned about from the wonderful queen of self-help, Louise Hay. Do this practice, this mirror work, every day for a month and you'll begin to start a whole new relationship with yourself.

2. **I sleep the best I can at night and make up for the shortfall with naps when I can** - Being exhausted and stressed has become an insane badge of honor for so many women. I used to be one of them. But I've made a conscious choice to eliminate that type of mindset from my behavior. There are of course stresses that we can't avoid and some stress, like good challenges that push us out of our comfort zones, are essential for living a full life, but the idea of crammed schedules with ridiculous hours, being ruled by social media and mobiles and commutes that eat up several hours of daily life have gone above and beyond what we

should consistently tolerate without question. "Busy-ness"
has become a kind of sickness. It's like the busier we can say
that we are, the more "special" and more "needed" by the
world we can feel. But the truth is that this enforced
busyness is bullshit behavior. It plays havoc with our weight,
our skin and our overall outlook. Sleep is a rejuvenator for
me and if I have to bring it back to my gray hair, nothing
makes me feel like I'm letting myself go quicker than
messing around with my sleep.

3. **I love my skin** - Just like my body, my relationship with my
   skin has become one of appreciation. Skin is insanely
   magical and the better I treat it the better it looks. And you
   guessed it, while of course this means to keep hydrated and
   nourished and all the things that we know that we need for
   good skin, I'm really talking about applying constant loving
   kindness to it. The nicer I am to myself when I cleanse and
   moisturize my skin, the more it instantly reflects that care,

not only in the mirror but in the feel of it. Being kind to my

skin, after all those teenage years of cursing it, has been one

of the most breakthrough beauty experiences I've ever had.

4. **Find A Style Spirit Animal -** This one is really helpful for

    me because I'm semi- clueless with fashion. I win the prize.

    If I had my way, I'd be wearing what I'm wearing right now

    as I write this - my uniform of my army cargo pants, a t-shirt

    and a hoodie but when I have to be real with style I've

    found icons that I follow on Pinterest and Instagram who

    match the look I like. And as much as I love Cindy Joseph

    and her whole vibe, my spirit animals don't have do the gray

    hair thing. I don't lock myself into the category so much

    that everything that I do is defined by that paradigm.

    Following fashionable women who I relate to helps me

    know exactly what basics I need to pull out as well as what I

    should take more risks with.

5. I stick with beauty guides that make me feel empowered, not enslaved - For me, the emphasis on beauty vlogs veers into old school tabloid magazine territory. I love that there's information, reviews, comparisons and previews of items that I'm looking for or things I need advice on - that's how I found the "co-poo" method of washing my hair - but my goal in life is having less stuff and that absolutely applies to cosmetics.

Lesson Learned

A practice of appreciating your inner beauty, never becomes an "empty"

Working the gray hair adventure in a way that keeps you feeling sexy and current means keeping a promise to yourself of working the inside as well as the outside. Know what makes you feel feminine and beautiful. Be willing to lift your game in a way you can live with whether that means trying a new lipstick color or wearing occasional heels rather than flats. But also be willing to work your beauty from the inside. Value every inch of yourself. Appreciate every opportunity your body, face and hair have given you. There is nothing else that will make you more beautiful.

SECRETS AND LIES

The weirdest discovery of my whole gray hair journey was when I hit the 12 week mark of no longer coloring. My gray roots sure didn't look the way they did when I was covering them up during my dyeing days. I was expecting a super distinct "line of demarcation" between the colored craptastic and the new grown hair. For many women this is the moment that lets them know they are really in the game. But for me, the result was surprisingly *underwhelming*.

Sure there was a fleck of silver, quite a few flecks actually, but here I was three months down the track, longer than I'd ever dared to wait between coloring visits and there was hardly enough to justify the mad panic of coloring appointments that I used to schedule on autopilot. It didn't make sense though because when I was still in coloring mode, the gray was definitely more apparent than now when I had given it up all together.

It made me wonder if our minds are influenced in a very secret, subliminal way by fear so that it amplifies a problem. For example, back in the day when I was routinely at the hairdressers trying to keep gray away, my mind and my eyes were totally primed to notice even the slightest hint of silver. Seeing these flecks set off a sort of alarm system in my head that there was a situation that needed to be dealt with. If *I* could see it, then the world could see it (and we couldn't have any of *that!*). But now that I'd reset my thinking as *choosing to see gray as a victory* and something exciting, my brain no longer exaggerated the issue or interpreted gray as an evil invader that needed to be attacked.

During the year I stopped dyeing my hair, my graydar honed in on anything gray related like a heat seeking missile. I noticed the media enjoyed keeping us primed to be on the lookout for stray grays at every turn. At the supermarket check out line, a tabloid would show a cover photo of the royal Kate Middleton holding

on to her baby with a heading "Has Kate Been Too Busy With

Baby George To Get Her Roots Done?" Or a link on a website

pointed me to an article titled ""Katie Holmes Reveals Flecks of

Gray. "Even celebrities who've *dyed* their hair gray for edgy

fashion or a movie role get coverage dedicated to it with online

galleries like "Stars Who Went Gray (On Purpose)" or "Julianne

Moore Goes Gray For Hunger Games."

Media gray shaming definitely plays a role in our paranoia over

our hair. It whispers that it's safer to keep dyeing than be caught

out. It's like when a paparazzi's lens zooms in on a celebrity's

behind in a bathing suit and acts like the cellulite on her

perfectly fine body is a crime. Like it's something we need to

know about! We get these messages and even if we don't go any

further than spotting the pics with a passing glance, they go into

a little pocket in our brain that keeps us on alert for these "faults" in ourselves to the point where being in our own bathing suit can feel fraught with danger.

But it's not enough for a pack of media wolves to make us feel fearful of gray. We seem to be completely fine as partners in crime when it comes to pushing along the fear and the myths about gray hair. Read any online comments on stories about gray haired celebrities and you get everything from blatant agism to mentions that going gray is fine for men and not for women. And by the way, have you ever heard a man say this? I sure haven't. In my experience, it's always a woman.

Why are we so eager to pass on fear of gray rather than challenge those who put that out there? Why are we okay with wanting to continue the idea that gray is only acceptable for men?

It's time to answer that question that I wondered about earlier. Are we women our own worst enemies?

Possibly.

Studies suggest women are tougher on each other than they are on men. Not only that, we're apparently the first to criticize and sabotage each other. Reasons why land between a tendency towards low self esteem and conditioned responses, to evolutionary explanations. We get aggressive towards each other because we're honing in on some primal desire to compete for limited resources. The caveman thing *again!*

All these possibilities make sense to me but we're evolving. I question just about all the "rules" now. When it comes to the one about men and gray hair, I actually use men with gray, like the George Clooney's of the world, as my inspiration to keep going with what I'm doing. The confidence and "no big dealness" that men have been allowed to have in the gray department, without all the loaded drama attached to it would be so freeing to have. I want a piece of that and so I take it. Dale's got that. He's been a silver fox for a while now and I love being in his club. All the things that they say about men and gray hair, about being suave, sophisticated and distinguished are fine descriptions to take for ourselves. And so I do. #ThanksClooney.

And what about gray hair on the job? Does it keep us from getting hired? Does it put us at risk of getting fired? During my research I read countless articles by human resource "experts" and employment agencies stating that women, and even men, should think twice before they allow themselves to go gray if they want to get (or keep) the job. There's no doubt that agism in the work place is alive and well and there are countless studies to remind us that things need improvement.

But here's the thing.

On a personal level, I'm self employed so my initial concerns about what this would look like for my work have vanished because I feel good and real in myself. For every woman I know in the corporate sector, not one of them complains about being forced to color their hair because they've been threatened of losing their job. In reality, no one is holding their feet to the flame and forcing them to dye their hair, except themselves. Continuing to dye is their choice. In fact, the idea that job advisors continuously push forward the necessity to do something extreme and even unhealthy for some like coloring, rather than focus on empowering ideas of staying relevant - in body, mind and style, not to mention job skills, is wrong. That we don't question this is even worse.

I think that if you're in a career circumstance where it seems the pressure is on to *not stop* dyeing your hair, even though you're desperate to do so, it might be good to ask the following

questions:

What other ways, besides my hair can I step up and be relevant?

Is the paranoia of not being who I am worth this particular job?

Would working in an environment more conducive to my

values be a better option?

What would happen if I back my choices and trust everything

about myself rather than buy into fear?

I *know* these ideas are easier said than done when you need to

put food on the table. In no way do I want to belittle the fact

that sometimes "you do what you gotta do". But I also think

that we deserve to get a conversation going about this and

admit that we play a role in continuing the madness of feeling like companies are coercing us to dye against our will.

I think group force might be the change for this. You'll recall there was a time when you couldn't have tattoos on the job and you especially wouldn't want to do an interview with them on display. This is one of those workplace taboos that's definitely shifted as ink's gone mainstream. Maybe as the numbers rise, gray hair might also be less of a target.

During my time on this ride, I came across a more poignant truth about gray hair. I was getting a lot of comments from younger women, under 30, who were going gray and even found their first silvers when they were teenagers. Going gray for these women is about genetics and I really felt for them. They were getting the ridiculous myths and fear mongering stories thrown at them, all for something that was completely natural. I felt sick at the idea of them spending *years and years* feeling afraid of being themselves. I was so moved I wrote this

letter to under 40's on my website:

Dearest You,

Last year, when I decided to stop dyeing my hair to let it grow out gray, I learned some weird things about us women. For one thing, I learned that the mere idea of publicly showing regrowth could put big time fear into the stomach pits of usually tough and independent women. I learned that to choose to grow gray is considered by some HR consultants as a career killer and I got the message that many women believe gray hair symbolizes giving up and everything bad about aging.

But the biggest surprise of all was hearing from you, women under 40 who were dealing with the same issues that my midlife peers were. The majority of messages I received this past year were from women, many in their 20's, who noticed their first grays as teenagers and now were in full "run for cover" mode. But the thing was, the women who wrote to me wanted to stop dyeing. They just had no idea how to move past the fear.

To tell you the truth, I hadn't really thought that this issue was a thing for women under 40. But the more I thought about it, the sadder I felt. I spoke to friends who admitted they'd been hiding their "under 40 grays" for years, afraid to tell anyone about it for fear that they'd seem old before their time. When you run the numbers, that's a helluva lot of *years* of fear. That's a huge chunk of time keeping a very personal secret.

I often wonder what's the price of fear when it comes to all this beauty stuff we feel that we have to do? Perhaps it's so many jolts of adrenalin that somehow impacts us on a physical level. Maybe it's missed opportunities to really see what our true, unique beauty would deliver if we let it. But these were thoughts that I mostly reserved for my age group and the choices we're making to keep that "50 is the new 30" thing, alive and well. To think that you, my younger friends, also go through this, hurts. It makes me feel like all the self acceptance and self love that we're trying to live and breathe is just a bunch of talk and something that really hasn't sunk in on a collective level.

And at the same time, I have a feeling that you're the ones that can actually stop the madness.

For one thing, the whiff of fear that you're getting is coming from us, the over 40 generation. Most likely you heard from a family member, an adult friend or the media that gray equals bad. Before the internet came, word of mouth was really all any of us could rely on – that's all we knew and so we had no choice but to keep dyeing our hair and passing along this misguided mantra. But that changed once we were able to go online and find others not only daring to go through the same thing but looking amazing while they did it. This was something we didn't really know existed and we started to have a change of heart. The gray hair adventure symbolizes a lot of the challenges that many of us over 40 face. A lot of the confusion is because the things that we were brought up to believe are no longer true. At the very least we're learning that it's okay for us to follow our own intuition rather than following the pack. But we're just starting to get this. Your generation however has got this way early on. You aren't confined to a lot of the ideas and mindsets that have brought us to life's crossroads. You might very well avoid some of the situations we find ourselves in now.

You learned early on the importance of being true to your soul's calling. It's normal now for us to talk about our purpose and many of you are able to express yourselves in ways that a lot of us over 40 are just discovering. You know how to be healthy and that it's more than what you eat – it's how you live, who you surround yourself with and what you do in the world. These are things that a lot of us at midlife are just wrapping our heads around.

I'm not saying here that growing gray hair is easy at any age, especially if you're young. Perhaps the advantage of being older and doing it is that the years eventually can provide strength and discipline to face up to what others think. But I do think that if any generation can turn our mind around about this hair thing, it's yours. I get so much inspiration from younger women these days. You seem so much more worldly and confident than

I remember of my generation. When I see a young woman who is letting her gray show through, I'm in absolute awe. I not only see beauty, I see confidence, I see style, I see someone who knows and backs herself 100%. There is nothing aging about that, in fact it's super human.

So, younger friend, if you're thinking about taking a break from coloring your hair but you get pushback from a parent or a colleague or other obstacles, know that out there, I'm cheering for you. You, being you, gives all of us, regardless of our age, the social proof that we can do what we want with our hair (our bodies, our choices, etc.) and do it without fear.

Some good questions to ask yourself are:

20 years from now, will the fear I spent not doing what I wanted to do be worth it?

What will happen if I see what my hair looks like without dye?

What will happen if I don't see what my hair looks like without dye?

Hang in there beauty. The lessons you can start learning now will make all the difference to your life down the track.

Love xx

Sue

As I write this book in 2015 the tide is definitely turning.
#Grannyhair is a thing. For this moment it's one of the the
hottest trends on Instagram and alive and well on the streets.
This year Amazon reported record breaking sales of gray hair
dye and *men*, wanting a piece of the "Clooney Factor", were
major customers. And most ironic, the same tabloids that were
happy to report about a stray gray coming out of a young star's
head now run stories about how gray is the new must have hair
color.

Go figure.

The trends might fade, but the gray hair adventure taught me
that questioning everything is forever.

Lesson Learned

Haters Gonna Hate But You Don't Have To

When I was a kid I used to love Roseanne Roseannadanna on Saturday Night Live. If you're around my age and from the States, you probably remember the comedian Gilda Radner's frizzy permed character who'd give consumer reports on SNL's fake news. Her signature line was "It's always somethin'." This comes to mind for me when I think of how we've allowed a kind of herd mentality to guide our choices about something as harmless as not dyeing hair. Unchallenged media messages combined with our own conversations have kept us afraid of something that maybe isn't even there.

It's always somethin'! There's always going to be something or somebody that's gonna want to challenge our choices. There will always be circumstances floating along in the ether that threaten to scare us. The gray hair adventure is the perfect

teacher for trusting yourself first. Bypass the comments of a one

sided tabloid story. Ignore the faceless responses that are more

troll than thoughtful. Tap into what's right for YOU and then

honor the answer. Your unique headline will be sensational, for

all the right reasons.

SURVIVING THE
WOBBLY MOMENTS

"Wobbly"

I was about four months into not coloring anymore. The new hair coming out of my head wasn't the harsh clash against the fried dyed strands that I thought it was gonna be. Let's face it. I got a serious pass when it came to the dramatic line of demarcation that so many women go through. I know that. Instead I was getting tinsel that seemed to blend into my hair and I was feeling pretty at ease about the whole thing.

But then this happened.

I got wobbly. Completely out of the blue. I was hit with the idea that maybe this whole gray hair adventure thing wasn't such a good move after all. More than that I got downright shit scared, a feeling which so far really hadn't landed.

The most obvious buttons in my psyche were getting a good pushing with questions like "Yikes, is this actually making me look like an old lady?" and "Is this gonna be a real relationship buzzkill?" All the stuff that I'd been constantly talking about challenging in others, I now was facing for myself.

The wobbles got me when Dale and I were on a vacation in Bangkok, Thailand, one of our favorite cities in the world. I was in the hotel elevator, doing the obligatory "check yourself out in the mirror" thing. With an overhead light that wasn't a girls best friend to begin with, I could see silver hair sticking out of my head like spark plugs. And I couldn't blame them on Bangkok humidity, this was all my own doing.

In the harsh glare of the fluorescent bulbs, the few flicks of silver looked more old and unkempt than a preview of something exciting to come. They seemed to emphasize the lines on my forehead. I couldn't blame those on stress because I was beyond chilled with all the holiday spa treatments I'd been having. *Pampering, shmampering.* There was no fooling myself. I looked older than I felt.

I wish I could tell you that I gave myself a wink and a smile when I saw this reflection. I wish I could tell you that I went straight into mirror work and told myself I was beautiful. But that didn't happen. In fact, the first thing that popped into my head was "Oh my God. What the fuuuuuuck am I doing?" It was almost a knee jerk reaction before I could lovingly talk myself down.

Clearly, this wasn't looking like I thought it was going to. There was no Cindy business happening here. No doubt at all, I wasn't growing gray hair, I was growing gray wires. Wires were one of the complaints that I'd heard from many women, like me, who were going into it with naturally coarse hair.

Part of me hoped that my hair would defy logic and emerge from my head a completely different texture than I'd produced before. But it was clear now that there was no denying it. Wires were going to be my fate. It wasn't the look I was banking on and here I was.

Now what?

My mind went from WTF to extreme self care mode and fortunately for me, it didn't take long to work this one out. I went straight to a hairdresser in the center of Sukhumvit for an emergency blow dry which in Thailand is about $10 including a tip. Note to the fellow sisters who have wires coming out of their heads, treating yourself to a professional blow dry, even at Western prices, can help get your equilibrium back after a wobble. It lets you take a deep breath.

In a modern salon with Hello Kitty décor, the hairdresser motioned me straight to the basin. The women that work there barely speak English but like just about every foreign place I've had my hair washed, the words "Blow Dry" transcend language barriers. As I followed her, I took in the familiar smells and sights of the salon. I realized that because I'd stopped coloring, it had been a while since I'd been in one and I felt a wave of nostalgia for the old days. It felt good to sink back into that ritual of it all.

But then I remembered Thai hair-washes.

Every Thai (and Cambodian, Laotian and Vietnamese) hair wash I've had has been notoriously strong. Keep that in mind if you're traveling there and want to get a little TLC. The gals *love* to get the bubbles and foam going so hard, literally scrubbing your hair against itself. They work your hair like laundry on an old timey washing board. And because I have so much hair, the process takes on a life of its own. You can practically design circus animals out of all the suds that multiply out of the scrubbing. You could fill a tub with the bubbles. Maybe you could even hire a nightclub and have a foam dance party. And once is definitely not enough. After the first shampoo is rinsed out, the cycle repeats itself all over again. So that's two full on shampoos with your hair scrubbed to the inch of its life.

It's safe to say they were going for the "squeaky clean" effect.

But during past vacations when I was still coloring, all I could think of was, "Oh my god, they're washing the color I had done just for this trip, right off the follicle!"

Things were different now. I didn't have to worry about that anymore. "Scrub away," I smiled in my mind to the hairdresser in the exotic international language of hair-care. Maybe she could scrub off some of the fried orange dye while she was at it.

The wobble was starting to subside a little. I thought of all the

times I washed my colored hair with shampoo for colored *and*

damaged hair and watched it fade anyway, effort and dollars

literally swirling down the drain. I hadn't realized it but it was

another one of *those hassles about maintenance* that weighs on your

mind in a sly and subconscious way.

When it came to the actual blow dry part, we had a little bit of

confusion. The young woman in charge of drying took a look at

my hair and crinkled her brow making motions about the top of

my head. I could see that she was talking about the grays that

were poking through. With a thumbs up and a smile I tried to

convey that I was okay with it, but that confused her even more

and she called over the manager.

"You have regrowth," the manager pointed to my hair saying in

Thai-glish.

"We fix?"

"No," I said with a Thai-glish accent. "I want to keep it gray".

Then I gave them another thumbs up, and left it at that. It was in the *way too hard* basket to try and explain my story any further, let alone whip out any pictures of Cindy Joseph on my iPhone's Pinterest account. The manager translated some aspect of what I said to the stylist and then left me, but not before raising her eyebrow and kind of shaking her head as though it made no sense. She probably just chalked it up to another crazy tourist.

Under the blasting blow drier, I watched my wires begin to lay flat and my horse hair morph into silk. The gray, while no more than a couple of inches of regrowth long, took on a more unified, metallic effect as the drying went on.

For a moment, I could see myself in the future. I knew in my heart that even with the wobbles and even though this was early stages, that I was doing the right thing. Not only because the color itself was looking better than any dyed color that I'd recently had, it was because the whole thing was such a novelty. Even though it meant having to be a little bit aggressive and saying exactly what I wanted to hairdressers, even though it meant having to go beyond language barriers and endure a little confusion and a raised eyebrow to get what I wanted, there was a part of me that thoroughly enjoyed the novelty of being different.

While I absolutely loved no longer having to care if what I had paid for was being washed down the drain what I loved even more was not doing the *same thing* as everyone else.

And this reminded me of my tattoos. I have two of them and I got them later in life. One is on the inside of my arm and is relatively hidden and low key. The second one though is on the top of my foot and I have to admit, it was one of those "seemed like a good idea at the time" kind of things! It's pretty damn huge. Sometimes when I have to expose it, especially in a formal situation, I feel wobbly because it looks kind of trashy. It's a big lotus flower but some people think it looks like a Canadian maple leaf. Ha! That part of me that was raised pretty conservatively can't help but wonder what people will think even though no one's mentioned it ever.

But here's the funny thing with this tattoo that kind of backfired. Underneath any misgivings I have about it, I love it. It's very "me". Okay so it's a little larger than I had planned and maybe I'd change the color or design to something more refined, but ultimately and uniquely, it makes a statement about who I am and what I love. In many ways this is what was going on with my gray hair at this tender stage, a fine dance between having something going on that people might not understand

and resulting in a judgment and being totally stoked that I was *not* following the crowd.

Don't get me wrong. Countering the wobbling feeling didn't happen overnight. It was still taking time to adjust to the reflection that I'd seen, almost like meeting a new version of me. I found that I'd be looking in the mirror a lot more than usual, tilting my head towards the reflection to see if any wires had settled down or to kind of get a grip on whether what I was doing was heading in any of the direction that I expected. It was like being a teenager and wondering if my boobs were growing. And maybe there were optical illusions going on between the collision of hair that was far less gray than I ever expected and the dyed parts that were just so damn straw dry. Frankly my hair was in terrible shape all together. In the bigger picture, I knew that for that reason alone it was good that I was taking a break from dyeing.

During this time, it was challenging to do the Louise Hay mirror work concept without throwing in comments like: "I love you Susan, I really do, but hmmm, I'm not sure what to think about this hair!"

I considered this better than nothing.

This is where having people on your side really helps. I'd ask Dale for a "hair update" knowing he'd see it as a sign that I needed some kind of affirmation that there was light at the end of the tunnel.

"So, how's the hair?" I'd ask him, bending down for him to inspect my fledgling "new born chick" roots. I'm not sure what he *really thought* but every time, he'd sweetly smooth it with both hands and say, "It's coming in nice. It looks good". The support of at least one person in your life, during any wobble, whether it's hair or a serious crisis, can work miracles. By the way, I still ask Dale for "hair updates" but now it's turned into a bit of silly fun.

The absolute worst wobbly moment that I had during this time was when fears about looking like hell and aging myself before my time really seemed to pile on me subconsciously.

I woke up in the middle of the night with a real pang of fear in my chest about the way I looked. We all wake up startled in the middle of the night over something that might represent a fear but never before did I do this over my looks and it really jolted me. Here I was, a coach who focused on helping women feel great about themselves and yet, I was doing the complete opposite thing. Even with my coaching training, I was freaked by these feelings of extreme insecurity.

I looked next to me for a reality check. I needed to ground myself. There was Dale with his arm around me. *Breathe. Okay.* I scanned my body and went to an immediate place of being thankful for everything about it, that it had been healthy and produced three great kids. *Okay*. I summoned up awareness of every great thing in my life til my heartbeat had softened. Eventually balance and perspective on all the insults and fear that had somehow made their way into my vortex eased. I asked myself what kind of message was trying to be sent with these feelings? What was lacking that I even went to this place?

The answer came.

I vowed that when the sun came up, I would start moving differently.

When I was reviewing my lifestyle during those first early stages of growing out my hair, I realized that I was being a little more sedentary than usual. I always practice yoga and I do a lot of walking but the gray hair adventure had coincided with a lot of new projects for my business that kept me at a computer nearly all day long and my walking had become shorter and more sporadic. My energy was depleted and when that happened, I knew that my self esteem and connection to what was important also dwindled. I knew that the best thing for me to do to counter these thoughts was to ramp up my movement.

This is the part of the book where I remind you that getting out of your chair and out the door is essential for the gray hair adventure. I'm serious. #Dontrollyoureyes.

Walking is one of the simplest and most powerful healing modalities on the planet. It's something I talk about all the time and have used throughout my life to make change. But I didn't consider that it could be a tool for gray hair wobbles until I thought about how it works. It brings oxygen and blood flow to all the organs, especially the brain and endocrine systems. Even

20 minutes of moderate walking changes brain chemistry in a

functional MRI.

I always feel taller and happier when I ensure my walking is in

order and knowing that this could really soothe doubtful

episodes of the gray hair adventure should've been a no brainer

for me. But what can I say? I'd been working so hard on trying

to get my business going that I found myself going into what I

call "nerdom" - a kind of underworld that other writers

probably understand. Writing is such a solitary business and it's

very easy for me to almost lock myself away to work. It took

this near gray hair-triggered panic attack to wake myself up to

the fact that I needed to take better care of my self-esteem by

changing my physiology with a simple 30 minute walk.

I can't express to you how quickly moving your body in the

form of an easy walk can settle a wobbly moment. It really

didn't take longer than a couple days of having some good

walks that I felt like I was coming back to myself again. I think the reason is a host of things, from the obvious benefits that walking brings to the more metaphysical explanation of your soul knowing that you're giving some tender loving care and rewarding you with well being.

And then there was the wobble elixir that brought logic into the picture.

I asked myself the simple question "Is dyeing my hair an option that is right for me?" And without any hesitation, the answer was "No way." I just couldn't go back to it and even now, at a stage where I've had a lot of time to get used to the process, I feel the same way.

Every now and then I get suggestions that I should highlight or lowlight. Maybe in the future I'll change my mind, who knows. But at my wobbliest and for where I'm at right now, getting even a smidge of dye is about as enticing as going back to waxing my labia. I've got zero desire of getting back on the salon horse, hoping and praying that the color will come out right or dealing with the impact on my hair. The silver might've been especially scary in those early days and doing it cold turkey, without any coloring to ease the transition might've taken a long time, but I'd passed the point of no return.

But that's just my story. I heard from women who were kicking themselves for giving into a weak moment and returning to dye. Afterwards, most of these women went through a wave of emotions about what they'd done, from frustration and anger to being overwhelmed. They'd gone to all this effort in growing gray and felt like they caved under pressure. Some admitted that it seemed to mirror other areas in their life where they didn't back themselves and chose to follow the desires of others.

This is when the gray hair adventure gets epic. I love when it exposes a bigger, more important adventure for us to tackle than just some fleeting beauty moment. For example, I could've taken my wobbly moment, had a freak out and just stayed stuck at feeling bad about myself. But by scratching the surface just that little bit, this wobble gave me some great messages. This was my chance to get real about reinforcing my self esteem during this new stage of my life. Even though I thought I was strong in this area, there was room for improvement. I also got the message loud and clear that as a new solopreneur, without my usual social structure of daily places to go and people to see, I had to find better ways to take care of myself and to keep to my aim of always walking my talk. For you, a wobble along the gray hair adventure might reveal that now's the time to start backing yourself more with your decisions or uncover better ways to treat your whole self.

If you happen to be one of those who ran for dye cover when a wobble set in, it's natural to feel like you've wasted your time. But I think it lets you go back into the gray hair adventure with a lot more confidence when you try again. You can go through this *knowing*, rather than wondering, that you're doing what's right for you, even when the wobbly moments kicked in. You've been there, done that. You know for sure what's right for you the next time around.

Wobbly moments happen whenever we're heading down an unknown path and in one of my gray hair videos, I used the metaphor of the gray hair wobble for hanging tough in uncertain times. It doesn't matter what the subject is - health, relationships, career, life purpose, whatever, most of us have been brought up with a "cut and run" philosophy. To actually breathe through a challenge and be willing to take a wait and see approach and to look for deeper meaning while we're at it is a new concept for a lot of us.

So my theory for this particular video was to reference other areas in our lives that we want to change but a wobbly moment happens. I offered three ways to deal with them that were 100% experienced and road tested by me. And what I love about these three ways is that they aren't just about the hair.

1. RECOGNIZE THE WOBBLY MOMENT AND DON'T BE SURPRISED BY IT - The first thing that I feel is important to do when you have a wobbly moment is to realize just that; *it's a wobbly moment.* When it came to feeling wobbly about gray hair, I was actually prepared for it because I'd heard about it on Cafe Gray. It would've been one thing if I woke up one day going "Oh shit, what have I done?" or "Why am I feeling this way?" But I knew full well it could happen, I just wasn't sure how I'd react once it did. But knowing about it lessened the impact. Knowing that there will be challenges and rough patches and detours

before you take on any big challenge is risk management and helps you get clearer on crossing the finish line.

2. WHAT MESSAGE IS THE WOBBLY MOMENT TRYING TO SEND?

When I was having my wobbly moment I was able to look beneath the surface. Was I really setting myself up for success with transitioning to gray hair or was there anything I could do to make this time better? When I thought about it, there were ways I could lift my game not only with the messages I was telling myself but also with some TLC and mindfulness of how I took care of myself during my business day. They were worthy lessons to learn and fortunately I was willing to receive them. Wherever you're feeling wobbly in your life, ask yourself, "What could this really be about?" and "What can I learn from this?" and "What can I do better?"

3. WOBBLY MOMENTS PASS -

Let's face it. Who likes feeling uncomfortable? We avoid it any way we can. When a gray hair wobbly moment hits, it makes complete sense to want to find an escape hatch *pronto*. The strangest thing for me is that the *super pangy* stages of the wobbly moment I had only lasted for a day or two. It passed. And I actually found sitting with the discomfort fascinating because it allowed me to recognize this was a feeling where I had a choice *not* to take an action. How many times in life do we feel a feeling and immediately do something, without even considering the option of wait and see?

If you're not sure about this, here's a science experiment. The next time you find yourself mindlessly eating, ask yourself if you're really hungry or if you're trying to eat yourself away from a problem or an emotion you don't want to feel. The answer probably is an eye opener. That wobbly moment is a powerful thing. Such is the trance of the wobbly moment that it leads women straight to the colorist or a DIY kit without even thinking that taking a little time out and some extra TLC is what's really called for. Reminding yourself that you're smack in the middle of a wobbly moment and that it will pass is an awesome bit of arsenal to have in your back pocket.

Lesson Learned

Take a breather before you make any decision (or at least hold off til you've had a blow dry)

There are very few important decisions that we have to make in an instant. It might seem hard to believe but even serious medical decisions can often be slept on, not only overnight but maybe even for months. We usually don't feel this way at the time because our back seems against a wall. Time is so precious and we sometimes feel that not keeping up with it will let others down or have us slipping behind.

The important thing to know is that the heat of the moment doesn't necessarily lend itself to good decision making. When we're in fight or flight mode, we're more apt to run to the option that's going to fix things right away. Fine for the moment but maybe not so great for the long game. When that moment of panic eases and you can see more clearly, you might find that there were actually more choices than you originally thought. Or maybe when the rush of adrenalin passes, you'll see you actually didn't need to take any action at all.

So, the aim, when wobbly moments hit in any area - from your hair to an email asking you for an urgent response to a life changing moment - is to take a deep breath and give yourself time to see the situation with as much clarity as possible.

NOT FADE AWAY

If I have one pet peeve about working in the over 40 niche, it's the often tossed around line that when we women get older, we become invisible.

I'm gonna come right out and say that I call bullshit on this! Women don't become invisible as they get older if they *stop* seeking validation from the outside world and stay visible to *themselves*. But still this message, that midlife and beyond "ghosts" us is *so out there* and so pervasive that it'll take decades of calling out to reverse, if that's even possible.

Let's face it, many of us have spent *a lifetime* of thinking it was okay to place our confidence and self worth into the hands of other people and other situations. And for many years we get away with it. For some of you, heads have always turned when you walked into a room. For others, doors have been opened and seats have been given up. You get that I'm talking in metaphors for all the times that we got that little bit of extra attention just because we were younger right? Or what about feeling better about ourselves because we're attached rather than single. We get used to our validation coming from randoms, rather than ourselves.

The feeling invisible thing is pretty much a reality check that it's time to start being visible to yourself. A lot of women honestly don't want to hear this. It means we have to roll up our sleeves and work on ourselves. Honestly, it's much easier to whine about feeling invisible rather than to take matters into our own hands.

So how does confidence tie in with the gray hair adventure? It's pretty simple. If you've done the inner work and you've got a solid foundation of confidence then chances are you'll have a base that's going to keep you steady and strong, even when you get the wobbles. Even when you have to *open a door* all by yourself.

If you don't have that base, even better. Why? Because if you're willing, the gray hair adventure can become the best teacher, not only helping you to build up your confidence muscle but spreading to other areas of life where it's time to start becoming visible, to YOU.

When it comes to beauty, confidence is everything. Dr. Vivian Diller, a former model turned psychologist shared a story that when she first booked with the Wilhelmina modeling agency, the founder, Wilhelmina Cooper, gave her an essential piece of advice saying, "The chances of booking work for us rises the minute you take on an air of confidence, no matter what you look like."

One of the things about gray hair that completely bewitched me was this subtle element of confidence that came out of the women on my Pinterest pages. There are millions of beautiful women out there but something about this group, who were purposely going against the grain and accepting themselves, brought out my own confidence about the adventure. Their gray hair didn't whimper "I'm invisible, no one's looking at me." Instead it seemed to say "Good luck trying *not* to see me!"

We have to see and acknowledge our own beauty and be proud and confident to try new things, sometimes without the applause of others. Seeking outside validation for our looks and for our worth is a losing battle.

Here's how gray hair will make you visible to yourself (I've road-tested all of them):

1. **Connect with your body** - If you feel insecure with your

incoming gray, and looks in general, this is a time to connect

with something, that has *nothing* to do with your hair. The point

of this is to amplify the connection between body, mind and

soul. One thing that consistently helps me cope with the

changes that happen to my body at midlife, including ditching

dye and accepting what that will look like, has been my yoga

practice. As much of a cliché as it can seem, the saying that

yoga brings you inner peace is true. There is something about

working with your body slowly and consistently that helps you

develop a compassion for your physical self.

Eventually this morphs into seeing that physical part of you as

just a part, rather than the whole picture. You learn that there's

more to you than just a bunch of body parts. When you

practice for a while you might do poses that test your limits,

some are even scary. Sometimes, the practices that I have are so

challenging that I know that there's nothing that's going to be harder in my day than what I did in the morning. Yoga has always been a way that keeps me incredibly visible to myself.

While yoga is my thing, it might not be for everyone. Pilates, ballet or Barre classes are other options that teach you to work with what you've got and to develop a strong metaphysical core.

2. **Learn to do things alone** - Constantly relying on others, whether it's for a second opinion or so we don't have to be alone is a sure fire way to dilute our confidence. Women who are especially vulnerable to this are those who are always overscheduled. It's the busy-ness syndrome. They're always with people, even on the weekends after a big week. While connection and friendships are essential, there's a dark side when it overtakes your personal space. If you find you tend to run away from yourself by staying busy with others, you probably know it.

My suggestion is to gently start dipping your toe in the water of solo acts. Simple things like seeing a movie or going out to dinner or to a museum. If you wouldn't dare do this kind of thing, that could be a gentle nudge that now's the time to give it a try. It's a small way to start getting used to your own inner voice, and to start learning how to deal with any created thoughts that are coming your way. For example, if you've taken yourself to the movies and you're imagining that people are thinking to themselves "Why is this woman all by herself at the movies?' you can use *that* as a point of backing yourself. You can answer back in your head by making a very definitive statement such as "I'm taking myself on a date" or "I love to treat myself to some time out." It's almost like a bit of a role play so that when you get wobbly over whether people are looking at your gray hair, you'll have experience in accessing an answer that you can truly believe in.

3. An extreme version of doing things alone is to travel by yourself - This is another thing that I've done quite often sometimes for work and sometimes for personal reasons like visiting family in other countries. When you travel alone you *have to* back yourself 100% whether it's deciding what to do each day, where to eat, where to sleep, how the money works, how to get by with the language and on and on. Unless you want to sit in your hotel room the entire time, there's no space for being wishy-washy about your needs.

Successful travel depends on confidence, especially for women. And the cool thing about solo journeys are that you either discover or get constant reinforcement about how smart and tough you are by yourself. You realize that you can trust your decisions. You can admire yourself for navigating a foreign map or for meeting new friends and having a great and unexpected night out. Creating an amazing adventure is like confidence *crack* and in many ways, that's exactly what the gray hair experience can be. It's a unique, journey where you have a choice. You can cower and wait for compliments or you can fake it til you make it.

4. Start challenging your negative self talk - This has got to be one of the most key ingredients to truly being confident. It's where the inside matches the outside by believing and backing who you are, what you say and what you do. But there's a kicker. A lot of us are in crazy deep when it comes to completely trashing ourselves. It's such second nature that we do it without even thinking about it.

Don't believe me? Try this.

Put down this book, set a timer and go about your business for one hour. Maybe you need to do a little work, make some phone calls, clean up or look after the family. But have your phone in your back pocket and mark down every time a negative thought about anything crosses your mind. Maybe it's a conversation in your head with someone who's "done you wrong" or looping over something you screwed up on. If you do that one or when self-talk is anything negative about YOU, you get to give yourself double marks. Woo hoo! If you're like most, you'll experience a very confronting situation that a lot of our inner chatter is incredibly critical, even abusive.

There's actually a dark pay-off for self-criticism. It completely clogs the pathway to the things we really want in life. Ruth Baer Ph.D. explains in her book *"The Practicing Happiness Workbook: How Mindfulness Can Free You From 4 Psychological Traps that Keep You Stressed, Anxious and Depressed"* that harsh self-criticism actually interferes with progress toward our goals."

The obvious question is how do we change this? How do we break the cycle of negative thoughts? Especially the ones that spin around the most vulnerable parts of our human existence; our looks.

I really wanted to know the answers to these questions for myself. As positive as I thought I was, I knew deep down that there was work to do. Self doubt was a thought process that was always just around the corner for me. So I took some specific actions for a few months to learn new ways to think. What I did *anyone* can do.

I began with the most essential thing and that's to get a handle on where my mind liked to go. I started sitting in silence purely for the purpose of understanding this.

I knew this wasn't going to be an overnight discovery or fix so I committed to doing it every day beginning with just five minutes for several weeks and then slowly increasing my current practice by one minute each month. I eventually worked my way up to 20 minutes which is what I currently stick with now and probably will for a while because that amount of time is perfect for my schedule.

Of course this "sitting practice" is really "meditating" but I think the word "meditation" conjures up so many confusing ideas that describing what I do as just sitting in silence does the job and is easier for others to try. There's no mantra, there's no mala beads to count. I just sit wherever happens to be handy, often at the foot of my bed, set the timer on my phone and watch what happens with my thoughts.

It was either a happy coincidence or totally meant to be that I started this sitting in silence experiment when I was about 10 months in to ditching the dye. And it should've been simple, right? After all I didn't have to do anything but just sit there.

Hardly!

I don't think I had been sitting for more than a minute when I started watching all these negative thoughts zipping through my mind like cars on the Autobahn. Reality collided with fantasy. My mind wanted to make shit up! It wanted to complicate things. It wanted to live in the past and in the future. Anywhere but here and now.

Rather than try and stop these racing thoughts (good luck with that!) I tried to be curious. I'd ask myself "Is this really true?" when something was super negative and distorted. I'd counter with some kind of kindness, like saying to the thought "You're not real. Come back to right now."

These sitting practices became a diffuser for me. They've taught me to question the thoughts that don't serve me and to work out where they came from. They soothe me and continue to remind me that life is good, even during challenges. I always finish sitting by taking a moment to be thankful for everything in my life and to acknowledge how amazing it is to be alive. I mean it every time I finish. It takes patience and dedication to do this practice but now it's become as essential to me as flossing my teeth.

I did some other things to reprogram my thinking. I listened to certain affirmation tapes over and over while I did mundane things like getting ready for the day or doing the dishes. I read motivational books. I listened to interviews and watched documentaries about the concepts of the thoughts that we think. It seems like a lot of effort but it was also interesting how life seems to get better when you think better. I smile more and people respond. I notice abundance more than focusing on lack.

And it made me wonder.

I somehow had resisted the concept of having a positive mindset as my natural state. It wasn't my fault though, in fact it's a primal response that's embedded in our cells. As part of that whole evolution thing that's continually cropped up through this book, we've had to be on the look out for trouble. When life was purely all about survival, thinking happy thoughts would *not* save our lives. And for that reason, thinking positively now almost makes our brains sweat. Reversing how you think about yourself takes time but it absolutely works. And if you're doing the gray hair adventure, this is essential medicine that's going to make the journey a pleasure.

I want to give you a couple of affirmations to use that can act like a melody to the times you feel great about what you're doing as well as those that can be fierce medicine when it goes wobbly. If these affirmations are just *too far out* for you, try creating your own. There are only a couple rules when it comes to affirmations and that is to keep them in the present tense and positive. State what you want and act as if. You know, the ol'

"fake it til you make it" thing!

Here are some gray hair affirmations to use that would be

wonderful to flood your brain with:

"My silver hair is absolutely amazing."

"My silver hair is evolving perfectly."

"My silver hair radiates gorgeousness and gets better every

day."

"I love how I back myself and do what's right for me."

"The world responds in loving ways to the choices that are

right for me."

Powerful statements right? But they also will easily become a

part of your mindset once you get going with them. Even when

I've had moments of feeling a little bit wobbly about my hair, these thoughts of love and affirming how good everything's

going to be are actually stronger than my doubt.

Affirmations can be used in so many ways. You can say them

when you look at yourself in the mirror. You can put stickies on

your fridge to remind you of how beautiful your hair is doing.

Schedule messages in your calendar. Find "triggers" on your

commute so that every time you pass by a certain spot, you

know it's time to say your favorite affirmation to yourself. I did

the stickies and to be truthful, at first it felt a little cheesy. But I

also used this resistance as proof that this could be a good thing

for me to do. And they work. After a while you won't even have

to think twice about bringing this kind of positive dialogue up

when you need it.

The one overall experience that I've had with growing my hair

out gray is that it's one of the BEST ways to learn how to not

only adapt and be present with our changing physicality as we get older but to also NOT see it as a negative. To me, it's like beauty in reverse. We go through a process of running away from ourselves and when we finally are ready to see our true, unique beauty, it comes. I honestly feel that now, in my life I'm getting closer and closer to who I am as a woman, who I am as a person and a soul. I truly have never felt more beautiful because gray hair shows me what happens when I drop my guard down and allow myself to be vulnerable. I can stop running from myself.

What if growing your hair out gray was actually an intense beauty power move. An opportunity to completely grow into a confident woman like never before in your life. What if, with time and new confidence, your beauty explodes even more, not because it's coming from the outside but because it's well and truly coming from the inside.

This is what beauty is all about. It's about the place in your soul that is perfection. A reflection of love, not fear. It's absolutely thrilling to think that with care of ourselves we can get to a place where we exude beauty straight from our heart and through our pores. I can't think of any other beauty related concept that's as strong as this other than putting ourselves through some extreme makeover. This is way easier. Gray hair has the potential to not only grow our confidence but it can completely shatter the myth that our beauty fades as time goes on.

Lesson Learned

Open your own doors because someone is watching you

No longer buying into feeling invisible means that you need to be willing to step up and see yourself. It means not waiting for others to give you their approval and not caring if you don't get a second glance. You're 100% here whether you think you're being noticed or not.

Often when I'm out with my daughters, they'll point out cool looking older women. They probably do this because they know my focus is with the gray hair adventure but the point is, they're looking. They're noticing the women who are owning themselves and walking tall. They stand out, even among younger women.

Speaking of my girls, I know as a mom that there've been times in their lives when they felt alone, when peers or friends or just this big world made them feel small. Thinking about myself as a young girl I can say that *for sure* I had those same kind of times when I didn't feel like I was being seen or heard. As much as it's easy to blame a certain age, it's lazy thinking. Feeling invisible isn't attached to a specific part of our timeline unless we choose for it to be. It's just part of the fragile and vulnerable side of

being human.

The women who were clearly visible to themselves, enough so

to catch my daughters' eyes, move in life like no one is

watching. They are just fine to open their own doors.

I AM BADASS

The whole "invisible" thing reminds me of all the uber stupid

words and phrases of midlife that we're supposed to swallow

hook, line and sinker. I don't want to get all political here but I

think it's important to start pointing these out because they're

such a part of our everyday speak that we don't even realize

how subliminally limiting and damaging they are. It's just not

enough to go through the gray hair adventure and defy the

physical expectations. That's all awesome, yes! But saying "I'll

do whatever I want with my hair despite what society says"

should be our tipping point for debunking all the hot steaming

piles of age related crazy that we're supposed to assume are a

given.

Here's a taster plate of some words and phrases that make me

yell at Facebook posts. #breathe

Crone: I hate the word "crone" - the New Age label for post

menopausal women who use their elder status as a passport to

wisdom and empowerment. Nice idea but shocker of a word! I

have friends in the business who are super earthy and really into

the concept of the whole "croning" thing. Drum circles and

chanting to the Dark Goddess are sometimes involved. Don't

get me wrong. I love me a drum circle! And if I happened to be

deep in a forest one night on a full moon and saw a bunch of

wild older gals in rainbow baggy pants, performing Pagan rituals

and dancing topless with abandon, I'd have no choice but to

stop and check it out (while hiding behind a very big tree). That

would be a bit random! But I can't relate to it for myself at all

and reject that just because my period stops that I'll have

automatic membership in that club. #pass

But here's what really happens when I hear the word "crone". I

get douche chills. I really do. It turns my stomach. It makes me

feel like someone invented it to really hammer home the idea
that age is gonna make us not only undesirable but someone to
be avoided all together. The full power of what a bummer the
word "crone" is to me is when it's connected with the haggard
archetype of an evil witch. A conjurer who's happy to keep the
wart on her nose and the whiskers on her chin while she casts
her spells on anyone who comes within ten paces. She also
always has crazy cat lady gray hair and for me dear reader, that is
a look that's a little too close to the bone.

Age Gracefully or **Age Disgracefully:** When I was growing up
it was the thing to praise older women who aged gracefully.
After a while, our boomer generation started to question that
(for good reason) and declared that we should now age, *ta da,*
disgracefully. At first it was kind of fun to see ballsy grandmas
jumping out of planes and whatnot. But then I thought, wait a
minute. Why is that disgraceful? Why can't a person do what
they want to do whenever they want to do it?

Gracefully. Disgracefully. No thank you to either one of them. Frankly, I'll age however I damn well please.

Telling people of a certain age that they have to behave a particular way is as ridiculous as saying that to any age group. Infants, tweens, millennials. We're all aging. We're all getting older. Regardless of whether we're in diapers or Depends. It makes no sense to tell any other demographic that they should do it "gracefully" or "disgracefully" so why have we thought it was okay that either of these are a direction we need to follow.

My bush logic on it is that as a society we just have no idea how to deal with older people. No clue. These labels maybe help us wrap our heads around this generation of mystery. Maybe if we can put them (and eventually ourselves) into a nice little stereotypical box we can handle the unknowns of it all better.

I think I have a better label to aim for. One that doesn't involve chanting around bonfires, knitting quietly in a corner or jumping out of airplanes. It's also age and gender neutral.

It is to become a total and utter badass.

Some people are born with it. Some just have to be ready to accept it.

About a year and a half into my dye free life, I was walking on the grassed area along the beach. I was thinking about how much I didn't care at all about what I'd done. It was exactly the same feeling as when you're walking around with dyed hair. It's not like you're obsessed with your dyed hair every second of the day. It's all of a sudden part of you. That's what my hair had become for me. Part of me.

It was a fascinating mental line of demarcation in itself. A divider between that old world of fear and uncertainty to an acceptance and a normalcy. But it was more than that. I realized that getting to this point was a milestone. I felt like a badass for completely backing myself. Regardless of trend or opinion. I just did what was right for me.

Being a badass doesn't mean having to ride a Harley or have tattoos (but it could!). Being a badass might mean you feel a little squirmy even saying the *word* badass. I know even I, of the truck driver mouth, was a little concerned that I might offend any conservative YouTube viewers when I made a gray hair adventure vlog called "Activate Your Inner Badass". I got over that concern quick enough. It was something just about everyone that commented could relate to and that's what I love about the word. It is everything. It is confidence. It is ownership. Being a badass is about backing our potential and not waiting for anyone to give us permission to explore it.

Most of us though have this image of a badass as being a trouble maker. We can mistake rebellion and thinking outside the square as not being a team player. That's where we get it wrong. Along with owning ourselves, being a badass means accepting responsibility for our world. It means being willing to drop our armor and feel things. Brené Brown, the epic researcher who blew the world away with her TED talk on vulnerability, describes the ingredients even further saying that the qualities of being "tough and tender" equal "badassery". We can use our badassness like an alter ego super hero. Someone who gets things done because she's the one to do it. She might be afraid, but that doesn't keep her from honoring who she is and what she's meant to do in the world.

Through my life I've always admired female badasses. My grandmother was a badass. She was the matriarch of the family, ruled her kitchen and could work a serious side-eye if someone said something dumb. I think she would've loved it if I was able to tell her she was a badass.

The female badasses that I look up to are usually pioneers, artists, performers and athletes. Your badasses might be from other walks of life. It doesn't matter. What they'll have in common is that they have an incredible self belief and work hard regardless of having obstacles thrown in their way. And best of all, I'm pretty sure they all believe they deserve everything they've achieved in life.

Here's my current list of top 10 badasses. Some are always on it, some I've just discovered or they've done something recently that moved me and made me say, "What a badass."

Dr. Christiane Northrup

Ronda Rousey

Tig Notaro

Sandra Bernhard

Lily Tomlin

Patti Smith

Roseanne Barr

Martina Navratilova

Jane Goodall

Tao Porchon-Lynch

It doesn't surprise me that my list contains a handful of women who have either experimented with natural gray or never dyed it in the first place. They're all incredibly cool looking in their own unique way, but it's not so much about the exterior, there's something very powerful that emanates from them.

So, what does it take to bring some badassness into your own life? Here are five ideas that might do the job.

1. **Gray Hair Is An All Access Pass To Badassness**: You don't have to do the gray hair adventure to be a badass but if you're on the path, remind yourself that you're a total badass for doing this because you're honoring what your mind, body and soul are telling you. This is a powerful reframe to the wobbles or to the phony baloney invisible myth.

2. **Badasses Walk Tall:** Sit on any bench and watch the humanity. You'll notice a lot of people walk through this world looking defeated by life. So many have shocking posture and a lot of it's preventable. If you don't ever think about your posture, it's time to. Even a short course in Pilates, ballet or yoga might give you enough of a check to

see where you're at and to know how to do it better. Walk

with your head up. Smile. Look around. Shoulders back.

You know the drill.

3. Badasses Don't Wimp Out: Today I had to make an

inconvenient phone call. I could've put it off or dealt with it in

an email. The person on the other end certainly was fine to play

it that way. But not making a move would've dragged out my

stress and this wasn't a situation where more emails made sense.

Making the call and getting it over and done with was the way

to do it. Going a little out of our way and dealing with stuff in

real time, versus running the risk of countless and confusing

emails, texts or tweets is a badass move.

4. Badasses Have Some Kind Of Personal Totem: If you're

not sure about the whole badass thing, get yourself a ring, a

necklace, a pair of red undies, *whatever.* Find some little thing, only known to you that when you put it on, you imagine yourself transforming into your alter ego which activates your inner badass. It's fun to play with this concept. I mix my totems up. Like through my life I've always had a pair of shit kicking boots. When I wear them, it's business time, people. I used to have this awesome turquoise ring that my badass grandma gave me. I called it my power ring. I gave it to my daughter when she moved overseas and now it's her badass superpower activator.

5. Watch a badass in a live performance: Every time I have the opportunity to see one of the badasses I admire in person, I take it. There is something so energizing and heart opening about watching a person who's dedicated their life to their art. Breathing the air of one of your favorite badasses, even if you're in a crowd of thousands is life affirming.

Lesson Learned

Words matter. Find the ones that are right for you

When you go through the gray hair experience, you learn that a lot of the phrases you've heard don't necessarily ring true. Some are completely off base. The great thing is that it can prime us for all the words and phrases that get attached to our attitudes towards getting older. Now, we know we have a choice. We don't have to accept every label. We can completely argue ones that are downright inappropriate. We can even invent new words that leave us stronger and more supported.

Use the gray hair adventure to ensure every "label" that comes into your vortex as something that's 100% right for you. And know, that when you do, you're not doing anything wrong by rejecting what doesn't work. You're simply taking responsibility

for yourself and activating your inner badass.

WHAT WILL THEY THINK?

The other day I had one of those times that I thought was going to be the hardest part about ditching dye. It was a "What Will They Think?" or to keep things simple let's just call it a "WWTT" moment. I ran into an old colleague waiting in line for tickets at the movies. I hadn't seen her since long before I stopped coloring my hair and now, here I was, nearly two years since my last salon visit. Girls being girls, there was every chance in the world that she might've thought I looked older.

Guess what? I am.

WWTT moments like this one were probably among the top reasons why I held back on no longer dyeing. I wasn't sure if I could handle the opinions, said or unsaid, by people who knew me. It was right up there with being worried about looking older and having crazy cat lady hair.

Chance encounters, reunions, weddings, funerals, birthdays...
the list of social do's and obligations is never ending. Reuniting
with people from our past, even in the most fleeting moments,
are constant underpinnings to our lives. In a perfect world,
these dots on our calendar would just be about warm
connections but in the back of our minds, they can end up
being a pressure cooker of worrying about how we'll front up.
Marta Wohrle, the founder of the beauty website "Truth In
Aging" described it this way:

"Here is the incontrovertible logic that if you wanted these
people in your life then you wouldn't need a party to reunite
you. Still, there is a gruesome curiosity that propels us to these
events. You will be scrutinized by people whose image of you is
frozen in time."

Curious that thing about wanting to stay "frozen in time." I

started reading blogs about attending high school reunions, the

big daddy of WWTT get-togethers. One woman explained that

at her 20th reunion, one of her classmates predicted for her that

the next time they'd see each other, at their 30th reunion, she'd

be the "The Person Who Has Not Aged Since High School."

Flattered at the time, the weight of the pretend award backfired

on her. By the time this woman's 30th reunion came around,

those words of being expected not to age were doing her head

in. The pressure of having to live up to some impossible

standard helped her make a decision. She didn't go.

Did she take her old school mate's words way more seriously

than intended? Did she miss out by not going? Probably and

maybe or maybe not.

But such is the power of these gatherings with our past. While I don't do high school reunions, we all have our own versions of the get-togethers that we do go to, that we have to go to. Forecasting what was ahead on my calendar got me wondering what friends and family would think about my decision and sometimes even talked myself out of stopping dyeing for the moment. I'd ask myself questions like "My cousin is getting married in six months time, what will it look like then?" or "How will this look when I do that job with my colleagues who I haven't seen in years?"

Of course, I knew there was gonna come a time where I'd have to bite the reunion bullet. It was just never gonna stop. And so rather than focus on any insecurity, I made a conscious choice to approach these events in a way that I'd never approached them before. Here are the tactics I chose, but I'll be honest, they are definitely big girl pants tactics. They require you to be living and breathing just about everything I've said in this book and all my work.

If you're ready to put on those big girl pants, here's what I decided about the "reunions" I would go to:

1. **I woke up to the fact that it was *completely okay* to look "my age."** I know there is a lot of yak about the idea of 50 being the new 40 and 75 being the new 50 but honestly, what the hell does that mean? Why do we have to put ourselves into age brackets? How about the possibility of me just looking good for me? I knew I was ticking all the boxes of my physical, mental, emotional and spiritual health so what more could I possibly do?! My take was that I'd commit to looking great for me and if I looked older or my true age, fine. There's nothing I can do about it. For me, this was a bit of a breakthrough.

Once and for all, give yourself permission to lose the worry about "looking' or "not looking" your age. The effort should go into looking like the best version of *you*. That's enough, whether you dye your hair, whether you're in the transition stage of gray or whether you're fully rocking it. This isn't as easy as it sounds I know because we have a lifetime of conditioning that we're not enough and that we should aim to look younger than we are. I get it. We glow with pride when we're still carded (not sure why that happens to me honestly, but I love it every time!) or when someone flatters us when we're with our daughters saying that we "look like sisters." Affirming for yourself fun things like "I am my own kind of hotness" or "This stage of life is perfect for me," can help ease you into a mindset of owning who you are, right now. And speaking of lines like "50 is the new 30", isn't it time to stop pushing these stupid old sayings along? The numbers are dumb. Neither age matters. Clearly no one's gonna do it for us though, it has to be me and you.

2. **What other people think of me is none of my business.** I know you've heard this one before and it sounds all nice on paper and stuff, but to actually have to *live it* and *breathe it* is a whole other story. What this classic phrase means is that if someone is going to be hating on my hair decision, when I'm okay with it, it's for them to deal with. I don't need their approval for something I'm doing that's 100% right for me. For many years, most of us have been led to believe that we must constantly be looking to others for approval of what to do in our lives. We might have felt pressure to get married so we'd be socially and culturally acceptable or we might've gone to a certain college or chosen a certain career to please our parents. For many of us at midlife, the concept of finally *not* having to take on board someone's opinion might initially feel like a completely foreign concept, but dang it's freeing.

3. **If someone crosses the line with a weird comment about your hair such as "it looks terrible" or "it makes you look older" or "what a mistake, you've let yourself go" this is your awesome opportunity to once and for all face the concept of boundaries.** It's a modern concept to know it's okay to tell people they're out of line, regardless of where they are on the family or friend food chain. If you've put up with weird family members who behave badly or are great at doling out back handed compliments, you'll know exactly when a boundary's been crossed.

So how do you deal with someone at a reunion who crosses the line? Chances are, they won't. Chances are, these are the kind of things we make up in our head. But just in case, make a commitment to backing yourself with the finesse of a diplomat. Aim for neutrality. Be Switzerland.

Here are a couple scripts to follow in case someone at a reunion says something stupid to you:

The family member you always try and avoid tells you that you look terrible. You say:

"Well, you're entitled to your opinion but that's rude so I'm going to walk away." (And then walk away).

Your sister says "Your gray hair makes you look older!" You say:

"That's okay, I'm older than the last time you saw me and I feel really good." (And then you walk away)

.

Old boyfriend at the 30th reunion dares to say, "What a mistake, you've let yourself go." You say:

"No I haven't, I take very good care of myself. Good luck with your life." (And then you walk away)

You can see that these are straight forward, stand up for

yourself reactions that don't ignite with drama or theatrics. I

admit, if you're not used to backing yourself, you might not

believe they can come out of your mouth. Role playing can be

really fun and helpful here. If you have someone who loves

what you're doing, ask them if they can play the dysfunctional

troll that you might see at a reunion and have them hit you with

their best shot. Practice responding back in a straight forward,

non-emotional way. And just as important, practice removing

yourself from the situation whether that's going to be to talk to

someone else, go to the ladies room or go and sit outside with a

glass of wine to revel in how cool you are. The more you can

literally say it, the more confident you'll feel if it actually has to

be put into play.

By the way, I highly doubt your old boyfriend will say that. I

highly doubt anyone will say these types of things to you but if you feel in the least bit concerned that there's someone in your crowd who's going to be a one percenter, consider this your ammo.

One thing that's really important to note though when it comes to boundaries is to be responsible and NOT get over the top sensitive if someone says *something*. The truth is some people simply have no social graces and really aren't evolved when it comes to expressing themselves. They seriously have no clue! But even with that in mind, I've known people who completely fly off the handle if they even *think* that someone's looking at them the wrong way. So don't go into a situation looking for a fight. Give people you're unsure about an opportunity to surprise you. And you know what, if you KNOW someone's gonna be a problem, just simply don't engage with them.

4.It's not about you. Oh, this one is a big one because it really taps into a subliminal place that those of us who have an ego and who like to look good might not have considered and it's that a lot of times, reunions, are *not* about us. When we go to a big fancy do, it takes effort. We get decked to the nines. Some more than others and I know for myself, somewhere in the back of my egotistical reptilian small brain is the idea that I'm going to stand out.

It's deluded on paper isn't it? This concept that even though an event such as a wedding is about *someone else's big day*, I'd go into it with the idea that actually, the spotlight would be shining on me. Now this is such embarrassing, crazy talk and honestly I never intentionally had this kind of idea in my head as I've always thought of myself as someone who doesn't like being stared at. Seriously, I'd rather hang out in sweat pants and bare feet than be at any event but I'm writing this because I think it's a place where a lot of us go. When we've actually taken time to get our glam on, we also assume that we'll be acknowledged for our efforts.

At least that's what I used to think.

When it came to the lessons you can learn growing your hair out gray, weddings were my biggest teachers. During the first 12 months of my adventure, I had two of them to go to. The first one happened just a couple months into it and even though I was excited to go - *love a wedding, love wedding cake even more* - I felt at first like my scalp was under a spotlight. But it wasn't. No one cared. If anyone had the slightest shit to give, which they didn't, I would've looked more like I couldn't be bothered booking in for a touch up versus intentionally going on some adventure. But even that made me feel a bit brazen because I was breaking one of my own rules! I was going to a fancy wedding and boom, I didn't get my hair done for it. Rather than feeling self conscious, I felt like the pressure of doing something

I'd been enslaved to in the past, was finally off me. I was beginning to feel I was owning what I was doing and it felt good to do that in a very dressed up crowd.

The second wedding on the calendar was when I was much further down in the journey - about the eight month mark. Looking ahead, I knew this was when I'd be in full transition mode. There was more at stake this time because I was heading back to California to go to my cousin Robbie's wedding to his long time boyfriend Jerry. This obviously was going to be a big moment for our family because California had just approved same-sex marriages. It was a way that we could finally celebrate with Robbie and his mom, my Aunt Sharon, who had been to so many of our weddings, baby showers and more. It was beyond awesome to finally have the roles of celebration changed and to be able to reciprocate what they'd given to me and my family for so many years of my life.

But I knew it might also be weird. My family doesn't mince words. Given the opportunity, someone would happily say "Girl what the hell are you doing with your hair?" Now, don't get me wrong, I'm sure I had an advantage over women who had very striking lines of demarcation between their dyed hair and their natural hair. My salt and pepper gray might've had me feeling vulnerable at times but it wasn't dramatic. Regardless, there was no denying that I was no longer coloring my hair, on purpose.

But then, I got jolted by the heart of the matter.

Newsflash! This wedding wasn't about ME! Robbie and Jerry were getting married. I was going to be able to share in the official joining of two people who loved each other. And it was even more than that. I was able to show my cousins how proud I was that they were pioneers in this new chapter in our generation's history. It was absolutely amazing that my family was going to be able to experience this and it made me feel

hopeful for my kids' generation and the generations to come.

So many things in our world, that made no sense at all when I

was growing up from not being able to marry who you love to

even the idea of having to dye your hair when you were

perfectly fine with the natural gray color that it was, were

completely falling by the wayside and the fact that this shift was

happening was huge. #loveislove

I also knew that it had been a while since I'd gone home to

Southern California where my family is spread about. Most

visits back home were quick dashes, just a few days in to check

on my parents and a brief visit with each of my sisters and their

families. Before I knew it, I was back in LAX customs, heading

home to Australia. It was getting harder and harder to connect

with my extended family and I realized, more than ever and

perhaps this is just one of those things that happens as you get to midlife, but I felt I no longer had the luxury of time. This wedding was the perfect opportunity to really tell all my family, but especially those I didn't see that much, how I loved them and to celebrate it.

Being content with having a happy time and telling people I loved them was certainly a huge leap from where I used to be when it came to going to events or weddings or reunions. There was no ego here and even though I was going into uncertainty with the way my hair looked and the way it would be received, none of that mattered because I took the *spotlight off me*. This wasn't about me at all. It was my cousins' day and I was going to go there 100% to celebrate them.

I had to wonder how different life would be if I went to all of those past events in my life with a lot less effort on trying to look a part and spent my energy simply being there, with the highest intentions. Maybe at the very least, I'd have had more fun rather than preferring to stay home in my pajamas. *Maybe*.

5. **Make an intention of what you want the event to mean for you**. When I went to my cousins' wedding I'd gone through a lot of the lessons I've talked about here. I'd done several gray hair videos so I'd literally talked my stuff through. I had my boundaries well in place. I knew how to respond if someone had an opinion about it, but at the same time I, wasn't feeling overly sensitive if something did come up. I was committed to having an "it's not about me" attitude for the whole trip.

Fact was, I didn't look that great at this amazing wedding. I arrived there straight from working in the deserts of the Middle East and I was pretty ragged and weary. My clothes still had sand on them. I had laryngitis. If ever there was a time I looked older, this was it, even dyed hair wouldn't cover it up. In another time, insecurity would've risen and I probably would've apologized profusely for everything about myself but this time, I pushed that aside, thanks to this crazy and deep gray hair experience.

Rather than cower, I set an intention to be happy, to tell my loved ones how I felt about them and simply own my shit! I had a lot to be proud of. I was a healthy 51 year old who'd just been doing some amazing travel in crazy countries, I'd written my first book and had been working hard doing what I loved. My husband and adult kids were all wonderful and thriving. And for something ballsy and weird, I wasn't dyeing my hair anymore. Life was damn good and had come about because of how long I'd been alive. I had this overwhelming feeling that denying myself the grace and benefit of all the years that I'd lived was actually a *horrible* way to treat myself.

So these two attitudes of being happy to witness this momentous occasion and to completely own my new grown up self were my intentions for the day. The power of intention, stating exactly how you intend to show up for life, is that it forces you to be responsible for your outcome.

And you know what?

The wedding was awesome. There was so much love in the room. I saw family and friends I hadn't seen for years and of course, not one person told me that I looked older. How could they? I was bloody ecstatic to be there.

And naturally, the gray hair wasn't even an issue. The only reason it came up was because of a conversation about my gray hair YouTube videos. But it just opened up a conversation around the table about the idea of it all together. There wasn't any judgment or angst about it at all. No sooner were we talking about it, we were on to the next bit of chat to catch up on *or I was eating cake*, one or the other.

So here's the deal. There will always be events in our lives that we have to get decked out for. And yep, they're probably gonna happen during some of the least convenient parts of the gray hair adventure. There are many ways to style your hair and work this look during these situations but the truth is, the real work happens on the inside. This challenge is an opportunity to once and for all get 100% real with your self. Owning who you are whether it's how old you are or just knowing that you're living your life, with all its hills and valleys to the best of your ability is perhaps one of the most beautiful things that anyone, including you, will ever see.

Lesson Learned

Leave your ego at the door and your sweat on the floor

How many times in our lives does our ego keep us from moving in the direction of our dreams? Probably too many. Look back into your past and think about how many times you held yourself back from doing something because you didn't think you measured up? What would've happened if this facade was dropped and we just allowed life to unfold?

The spiritual teacher Marianne Williamson has a wonderful quote explaining what happens when we allow our truth to speak for us, rather than giving in to the ego's relentless need to be heard:

Ego says, "Once everything falls into place, I'll feel peace."

Spirit says, "Find your peace, and then everything will fall into

place."

These are simple truths. Nothing changes unless we do.

Nothing makes us happy unless we choose to be happy. We can

choose to put these concepts into practice or we can choose to

stay stuck in a time warp. Making peace with ourselves,

becoming our own best friend through every stage of our life is

what makes a reunion, a wedding and all of life's gatherings,

something to truly celebrate.

LE SUCCÈS EST LA MEILLEURE VENGEANCE

It had been about a year of growing out my hair gray. I was in a bathing suit store trying on a bikini. The light was incredibly unflattering making one of those *trying on bathing suit times* more loaded with the potential for criticism than usual. Fortunately, I'd been spending the months before really walking my self talk and thinking a lot about never criticizing myself for my looks. I knew that regardless of the way my skin looked in the harsh lighting I was super healthy and spent hours practicing yoga and walking. My body was just fine and even though there was a part of my mind that wanted to argue about that, I was able to completely override it.

In fact, while I bypassed my body issues, I noticed that the harsh overhead lighting actually was my hair's best friend. My silver could give Clooney a run for his money. It was Pinterest worthy! Usually my hair seemed to be doing a brown thing with wayward silver strands, but this time, under the ugly lights, it was bringing it. Back in the day, I would've paid for this gunmetal color.

I noticed that all the new hair was in such better condition compared to the straw tips that still hung at the end of it, my version of the ombre style. The difference between the old and the new was happily shocking. I almost had to pinch myself. I was finally seeing this new version of me. Here I was 52, in a dressing room trying on a bikini. Here I was in a dressing room with harsh lighting and being completely stoked seeing my hair silver. I felt like I was at the beginning of a journey, almost as though I was a 21 year old with my whole life ahead of me.

For that past month my husband and I had been changing the way we'd been eating. He'd been in a really tough work situation and the stress had taken a toll on his health. Finally, something gave out in his stomach and when everything escalated into a CAT scan (which in turn resulted in something that was vague and the doctors could give us no direction on) we immediately changed his diet and I was happy to join right in.

From the time I'd stopped dyeing my hair, I started slowly, slowly looking at other parts of our life where we ran around with our heads in the sand. Whether it was the crazy chemicals that were on our lotions and soaps to all the pervasive crap that was in even supposedly "healthy" food, I felt willing to open my eyes even wider than I thought they were. And let's face it, no one was going to do it for us.

We started very basic and just looked at everything we were eating and asked a simple question: Is this the best choice for us? The first place where this was an obvious "no" was with wheat and gluten products. Bread, pasta, bagels, etc. were staples of our life and had been for years. They were the bulk food that filled our kids up when we all lived together. But looking at them now just annoyed me. I had no idea where the grains were coming from or what all that wheat and gluten was doing to us. So bread, such a massive part of our lives, went.

Then we stopped with dairy, I'd given that up a while ago, but this was new territory for Dale. We replaced milk for coffees or cooking with homemade almond milk or coconut milk. We used the pulp from the almond milk we made and processed it into our own flour. We stopped with refined sugar and made our own deserts out of superfoods like cacao. Coconut oil took center stage for our food and our skin. It was a huge shift in a very short amount of time but sometimes, all it takes is a big reality check like a doctor's visit to shake you into action.

There was something different about changing the habits of our lives now. Besides that, there are so many great recipes online that showed me we could make these changes and gain taste experience rather than lose it, no longer dyeing my hair might've acted like a subtle domino effect. I'd learned first hand that the world didn't fall apart when I decided to do it. In fact, a lot of what I'd heard about giving up hair color didn't happen to me. It reminded me to question everything that we think we "have" to do. I'd grown up thinking that grains and dairy were essential, part of nutritional requirements. Perhaps they were in another time and place but now with the information coming out online, we couldn't ignore that sticking with these things, just because of what we'd learned decades ago, wasn't the most evolved choice.

After only a few weeks of this big swap in our food mentality, Dale and I noticed a difference. We were eating really delicious food and we were really excited about discovering new ingredients and finding substitutes. I was just as excited to be happy to be back in the kitchen. For the past few years, I found I was completely *over* cooking, I'd simply lost my joy for it. But now, I was interested again.

Dale's weird stomach thing vanished without any medicine or further doctor's visits. He lost 10 pounds without any effort and while my weight's been the same for years, I felt energized and excited by the concept of having choices in so many areas. And to fast forward a bit, this is how we eat now about 80% of the time. The remaining 20% is for when we travel, are socializing or occasionally craving something at home.

But back to those early days relearning how to eat, there's one particular weekend morning that you'll want to hear about. It was a typical Aussie summer Saturday. Dale had already had about three surfs at our local beach before breakfast. While he was out, I did my yoga practice. Back together we had banana avocado smoothies and got dressed to take a walk around our neighborhood.

A hair report! This was one of those days where even in the high humidity of the Australian summer, my hair, with about 2/3rds of it dye free was behaving itself. I noticed this because for years with my dyed hair, Sydney's humidity was an enemy for me. My hair would get so ridiculously frizzy that the only way to tame it would be to damage it even further by running a hot iron over it to smooth and straighten the frizz. Or I'd simply give up and twist it into a top knot. But on this day, all the myths about gray hair being coarse and wiry were simply not true. My hair, at least the gray part looked soft and interesting and even the usually dyed part seemed to be cooperating. #miracle

We walked over to our local surf shop. I was looking for some board shorts that I could do yoga with and then jump in the ocean after class. Our local shop is a total hangout for great surfers and while Dale was buying my shorts and talking waves with the owner, I turned around to check out some of the clothes. And who do I literally bump into?

The French hairdresser who told me my hair was going to look like shit. The hairdresser who I had fired.

I'd seen him a time or two over the year because he was a local surfer. It was fitting. My hairdresser walk of shame. Once was right outside my apartment on his way to the surf and we just exchanged simple but awkward "hellos." The other time was when we were at a show to celebrate local artists. Of course everyone in town was there and so was he. Again, it was weird with nothing more than a "Heyhowyadoin'goodtoseeyougottarunbye." We both knew what was up.

There was supposedly another encounter, but I wasn't there. At a party, my daughter Presley apparently gave him a cheeky tongue lashing about what happened. It went down in front of other people and she supposedly didn't hold back.

Ahhh, the joys of a small town and a daughter who doesn't think twice about speaking her mind. I felt a bit for the guy but of course I secretly loved that Presley didn't like anyone telling her mom that gray hair was a bad idea and she wasn't afraid to let them know.

But here we were, a year later. Face to face without any distractions to avoid a chat. Not only would it be uncivilized to not have a little conversation, in a weird way it was almost destined to happen.

We said our initial hellos and he told me that he'd opened a new salon in another suburb that was doing really well. We spoke about my daughter Presley and the shade she threw at the party.

She'd since moved to Chicago and was experiencing her first winter and snow.

We said just about everything there was to say and then finally it was my opening to bring out the gray elephant in the room.

"So," I said pointing to my hair, "Remember how you told me it was gonna look like shit?" I smiled, nodding my head down so he could inspect my scalp. And he laughed and in his thick French accent he said, "I know, I know and I have to say, eeet looks really cool."

"See...... I told you," I laughed, but then I added, "I'm glad you have proof that it can be okay."

We spoke for a little bit about hair stuff. He thought I had about two or three cuts to go before the dye would all be out. He passed me his card and I mentioned that *maybe* if I could ever make it to his suburb then *maybe* one day it would be nice to come see his salon and get a cut.

I mean after all, he did give my hair an excellent hair cut.

We said our goodbyes and the dust was cleared. It's funny too. It just seemed incredibly destined for a reunion between us to happen this way. It also felt good to have a kind of closure on a relationship that ended weird. This is regardless that it was just a hairdresser/client relationship. There's something that's always uncomfortable with sketchy endings and while I'm 100% for having boundaries and not needing to explain, there are also times when people evolve and when new conversations can be had.

Meeting the French hairdresser and getting his approval really wasn't about the idea of "success is the best revenge" although let's face it gals, this one felt pretty sweet. But the thing is that's an egotistical was of approaching it. The truth of the matter is that educating the mind to see gray as a beauty move rather than as a huge mistake that's going to be full of regret, can take time. It isn't just about hairdressers either. This scenario can happen with a partner, a family member or a friend who finally sees the light. Sometimes these things just take time.

And what I really loved about my reunion experience with this hairdresser is that I was reminded that sometimes others also need time to process what we're doing and come to terms with it. I mean let's face it, we spent time getting on board with it ourselves, by the time we tell people, we're way ahead. It was great to be reminded that sometimes we have to wait for people to catch up.

So would I have done anything differently if I knew in the end that my hairdresser and I would finally be on the same page? No, I wasn't rude at the hairdressers. In fact, he was out of line with me and I took the right action that we should take with anyone in our life, whether they're an authority figure or a stranger. *If you don't treat me respectfully, then I won't engage.*

But....

We also have to give the people who are unsure about our decisions a break. Going gray on purpose still isn't the norm and although it might be fun to say that gray hair is the new black, only a very small segment of the population would agree. The majority, even those close to us, need solid proof before they jump on a bandwagon. This brings up two things: when you're sure about something but others aren't, be willing to back your choices regardless *and* do that with the knowledge that some things are not an instant convince and take time for others to understand.

Lesson Learned

We're all doing the best we can

The French hairdresser reunion was symbolic for relationship challenges in general. All of us really are doing the best we can and we come at challenges, new ideas, and new directions with different thought processes. In my hairdresser's defense, he was young, only in his mid 20s and wasn't aware of a movement to stop dyeing hair. Maybe it just wasn't his thing and didn't need to be because clearly, his other clients didn't want it. Perhaps it would take countless Cindy Joseph wannabes to come to him before he could get on board with it.

Or maybe that would never happen. Who knows?

The bottom line is that we have to be *willing* to give people the same opportunity to change that we expect them to give us.

REGROWTH

The week after I had that random *but destined* reunion with my ex hairdresser it was time for me to post a gray hair adventure video. My inspiration for them always came from something from real life, whether it was something that happened to me or something that someone had asked advice on.

I knew that I needed to talk about the hairdresser because in my first video, I'd pretty much slanged him. It was similar to how I wrote about him at the start of this book. I knew that he was young. I knew he was a guy with bravado but it irked me that he didn't see where I was coming from. I always kind of felt that if this was happening to me, this was happening to someone else and it just seemed important to have my say about it.

I'd been doing the videos monthly for over a year. My feeling about the adventure was changing. In some ways, I kind of felt over it. I had gone from so many stages such as the excitement and wonder of doing it to the vulnerability of whether I would still be loved and feeling wobbly to what kind of hair products would keep down pesky wires. But somehow, over these past few weeks, my feelings about what I was doing started to fade into the back of my head. My hair, even though I still had another year of growing it out before it would be officially done had become *a part of me*, not something that was *defining* me. I don't know if this is a stage where all women who grow their gray hair out land but it's similar to all the things in life that at first seem very important and then we get use to. We get used to being a mom or not having kids. We get used to being single or being in a relationship. We adjust and we move on to the next thing.

But that meeting with my hairdresser got me thinking on a lot of different levels. That I got a chance to "prove myself" to him was the farthest thing from my mind. Actually, reflecting on the

SUSAN PAGET

past year, I felt like I was the one who had a lot to learn, especially when I started. In many ways, if I could've re-done my reaction to what had happened with him in that first video, perhaps I might've.

I started creating a video about the lessons that this hairdresser had unknowingly passed on to me. As I started to bullet point out what I'd learned, I actually felt quite humbled. This guy had inadvertently made me a better person. Without him, I wouldn't have been given an opportunity to dig deep and to feel vulnerable to the opinions of others. If I hadn't sat in that chair, I wouldn't have had anything to kick me into action to start documenting what I was doing or looking deep and trying to find meaning, behind the surface beauty parts of going gray.

I realized that through the past 12 months of the gray hair experience that I had really become so much more quietly confident than I ever had before. I felt beautiful. I felt strong.

I'd pushed through squirmy feelings and learned to enjoy being out of my comfort zone. And age had nothing to do with it. These kind of feelings don't come from getting something handed to you on a silver platter. From the start of the adventure I had to work for them whether it was getting over the feelings of vulnerability and questioning what I was doing to actually doing the grunt work of making videos, podcasts and writing about it.

Through the gray hair adventure I met really cool women who were going through their own. Writers, vloggers, bloggers, nurses, foodies, designers and more from all corners of the globe. I met women having victories and others who were just holding it together. For all of us, gray hair was really a symbolic thing for the other major stuff in our lives. All of us were just trying in our own little way to be authentic, be loveable and be ourselves, even if it was a little bit scary to go against the grain.

I never in a million years believed that I'd have a connection with online people but this thing, this gray hair vulnerability seemed to cut through any cynicism that I felt about the online world and brought the kind of connections that people can really have into a whole new realm.

When I looked back at the first video that I did where I explained my initial experience with this hairdresser I have to admit, I don't come off very well. Besides that, I was inexperienced doing videos, I feel like I come off a little too intense and indignant about the whole idea that someone (the hairdresser) dared to tell me his thoughts.

When I compare what I looked like then to what I look like now, I'm confident in saying that my dyed hair didn't suit me at all. It was a reddish orange that just had a hard look against my skin. It looked harsh, maybe I even look frightened, at least that's the subliminal thought that I have when I dare to watch it back. #cringeworthy.

In the videos that were from a year later, I know I was feeling more relaxed and at peace with what I was going through. In one of the later ones, my hair wasn't blow dried and managed. It was actually a little too long and kind of verging on wild, but something in me had obviously changed to the point of a very noticeable difference. Is it really possible that the simple act of growing our hair out gray can actually lead us to a place where we become a completely different, settled person who's more comfortable in their skin? If these videos were kind of a tale of the tape, then the answer, at least for me, is yes.

Despite all this video regrowth, I have to admit, I always was certain about what I was doing. I knew that even if and when it got tough, that it would be worth it eventually. I think that if there's any kind of advice I can give someone who is thinking about doing the gray hair thing is to wait until they get to this place. It's a place of knowing and of really being so certain that nothing is going to shake you. It takes a lot of thinking about it but you can absolutely feel it in your bones and in your soul when it happens. It's how it should be with any heavy decision in your life or any time you're trying to find a direction to head in. You know what you love, go there.

The year reminded me so much of the power of slow change. As I write this my hair still isn't fully rid of the dyed bits. I could cut them off but I need to wait another inch or two. It's a girl thing! I had no idea how long a month, six months, a year, two years is when you're waiting for something to specifically shift. There are a lot of ways to push it faster along, but the slow way for me was the right way. That slowness let me take on other challenges that forced me to be still with my thoughts and actions rather than act fast. The experiences strengthened my boundaries muscle and I learned how to say "no" to situations that didn't serve me, whereas in the past I might've said yes.

The irony that it was the hairdresser, who first completely was baffled by my decision to go gray but would indirectly become a profound teacher, wasn't lost on me. I thought when I sat in that chair that I knew everything about where the journey would take me, but in reality, I had no idea.

Lesson Learned

The more I learn, the less I know

What would happen if every time we're dead certain about something, we take a moment to consider that there might also be an element of mystery. If we don't, there's a good chance we really don't know what the hell we're talking about.

It's a scientific fact.

Known as the Dunning-Kruger effect, people who think they know a lot, tend to actually know less than they think. Psychologists David Dunning and Justin Kruger tested subjects on logical reasoning, grammar and humor and then asked them to estimate how they did. Those who scored the lowest were the ones who completely overestimated their results. It's the "ignorance is bliss" thing. Once we start the real learning of something, we soon see that we've actually got a long way to go.

For the gray hair adventure, it's essential that your doubt doesn't exceed your confidence in what you're doing. That's true. But remember, that along the way, even confidence can't predict the lessons that will be waiting to find you.

OUT OF THE CLOSET

"Hello everybody," Cindy Joseph's voice says from behind a sheer curtain hanging above her. She is talking to her followers in a video titled "Revealing My New Hair."

"I have a big surprise for you."

The curtain drops. Cindy Joseph's long hair is gone. The flowing angelic *young* hair, of silver and blacks, grays and metals, the holy strands that made up her signature mane and was so perfect that it almost seemed too good to be true, actually was just that. Too good to be true.

They were all extensions.

"Here it is. I took out my extensions and this," she said drawing a breath, "'is my real hair."

Let's be clear. There's really *nothing* that Cindy could do to make herself less beautiful. She's an extraordinary person, it seems on the inside as much as the obvious outside. But the Rapunzel-esque locks that got me over the line to do my own gray hair journey without a second thought were gone. In their place was a short, stylish bob cut to her jawline. The color was white veering into a little color texture in the back. But the complex layers of hues and bounty of curls were no more.

It must've been a very intense moment for a model to reveal herself without the look that got her jobs in the first place. Just like me, there would be a gazillion gray hair adventurers all over the world who would've used Cindy as their poster girl for all things gray and she would've known it.

To her credit, she didn't keep the extensions that she had a secret. I'd heard her mention them in a past video but I didn't pay much attention since extensions are like Hollywood tape

and wind machines for models and celebrities. I just didn't
grasp the extent.

At first, I was confused. The irony of it all hit me. Just like we
flock to buy the latest anti-aging make up's and skin care lines
promoted by airbrushed actresses who swear they don't use
Botox, fillers and everything else, this low key, but glamorous
silver haired goddess was also a part of the media machine to
keep us lusting for something that wasn't real. Who knows,
maybe this look wasn't even possible!

And then there was the second irony courtesy of all people, the
bloody French hairdresser!!!! The gift that kept on giving!! My
mind rewound to that day in the chair and my last ditch effort
of getting him on my side about ditching gray. I'd pulled out my
iPad with all those *Cindys* smiling up at him to which he'd
barked, "Photoshop, make up! Eeets all bull-sheeeet!"

God damn it. He was right.

I'll have to tell him about it one day. #FairsFair

I'm gonna come clean with Cindy's video reveal. I had to process all *this*. It was a lot to take in! I had to completely get over myself before I could really appreciate how damn hard this would've been for her. I got myself together and started to listen.

In the video Cindy told the story of how she came from a family who genetically had very fine and thin hair and that she never felt good about hers. As she told her story, my heart opened.

"My entire childhood I was told, 'thick hair is good' and I tried *everything*, hair thickener, permanents...any new product, I tried."

I've rewatched this video several times since that first time, in fact it's playing in my headphones now as I write and it continues to move me. As composed as she was in telling her story, I can totally feel the agony of a young Cindy thinking that she wasn't *enough*. She grew up *believing* her hair was "defective" and "wrong." That's a lot of belief to carry around as a young girl into forever.

Her words transported me back to those frustrating years of mine as a self-conscious teenager trying everything under the sun (often literally) to make my skin normal, like everyone else's. I absolutely felt defective and wrong. I'm sure you can relate to what she's saying, even if it wasn't your hair or your skin, there must've been something that got you down as a kid. But the thing for me with my skin was that I grew out of it *eventually*. I know that the experience has left me mindful but I was able to see a light at the end of the tunnel. And I certainly wasn't a model! Between never getting a reprieve from something that I couldn't help to having to make a living based on it, I would've lost my mind! That kind of never ending insecurity would've been a horrible weight to drag around.

Cindy told the history of her extensions, explaining that she lived with them for 14 years encouraged by hairdressers who wanted it thicker and longer and all the things that she naturally wasn't capable of. Understandably, after a lifetime of feeling ashamed and insecure about her real hair, she wanted it that way too. She had fun with it.

Things changed recently though. When she started her cosmetics company aimed at making women feel good about aging, she admitted she started to feel like a fraud. She knew that she finally had to, not only make peace with her baby fine hair, but to love it. The weight of her responsibility as this unofficial hair role model also fell on her but not in the silver hair way that I thought. She explained that what got her the most was knowing that women around the world, who had thin hair but were seeing her many photos, and wishing that they could have "that" was something she could no longer live with.

The word "fraud" is something I can sometimes relate to on this gray hair journey. While maybe Cindy's hair was too good to be true, my "gray" hair sometimes can't even be called "gray" and here I was making videos about it and writing a book about it. My hair didn't go the full silver I expected. It's a salt and pepper, the kind of salt and pepper that a lot of people don't even like. Sometimes, in certain light, you can barely even see any "salt". It just looks brown.

Lying in bed some mornings I ask Dale that old funny question of "How's the hair?"

"Fraud!" he jokes back.

It's funny how *even in doing the gray hair thing*, we can have moments where we don't measure up, where we aren't enough. I used this as the inspiration for one of my video updates where I sang a song, inspired by Cindy's perfect hair, that went "Am I not pretty enough, if my gray hair ain't like Cindy's...."

Sigh.

Throughout my time on this weird head trip, I've talked to women who've felt bad about not being able to ditch dye. Seriously, they really get upset about it. It's something that they really want to do but they're just not ready or they're certain it's not going to look good on them. This loony peer pressure has probably come about because of all the images, videos (mine included), sites and movement in general to embrace gray. But there's also a tendency for this gray hair adventure to become almost militant and judgmental about women who do dye. The wrong message that seems to be coming out is that if you don't join in, you're unevolved.

That's so unfair and so untrue. All of us deserve the right to feel pretty and feel okay with what we're doing. More than that, we all deserve to have a choice. That's all. And let's get real, can you imagine anything more boring than having *everyone* walking around with gray hair? #nothankyou.

As the video went on Cindy explained that everything was pointing to parting ways with her extensions. Her friends wanted them out. Her husband begged her to do it assuring her that he loved her, regardless of how many hairs she had on her head.

Before she did the deed, she called her booking agents to tell them that she now had short hair. She found a supportive hairdresser who would take her through the process slowly and gently and then give her a cut that would make it look healthy.

I've kind of fallen in love with Cindy all over again. She's still my Queen of the Silver Sisters but now she's more than a cut-out paper doll for grown ups. Maybe we needed someone like Cindy to get our attention and wake us up from the coma that we had no choice. Then, once she had us she could really tell us the truth about beauty, how the surface stuff is nice but there will never be a substitute for loving who we are and the goods we've been given through every stage of our lives.

"So, here I am," Cindy said, looking down the barrel of the camera. "This is me."

Lesson Learned

Look beneath the surface

We live in such a fast and noisy world that it's easy to completely overlook the heart of what's out there. If we don't like the look of something we move on. In my case, it would've been so easy to spend five seconds on a model's video, check out her new look, make a judgment and move on. But if I did that, I would've missed the hugest message. Not allowing ourselves more than a moment to understand what's really going on might seem convenient at the time, but we lose in the long run. We miss out on some of the biggest and most surprising lessons of life.

The deceptive part of the gray hair adventure is that on the surface, it wants us to just look at the hair. It wants us to only care about the style or figure out how to manage it. We think for it to work, it has to look like an impossibly perfect picture on a Facebook page. That's the aim, but it's shallow.

It misses the point.

Look beyond the superficial. Whether it's not dyeing your hair or making a major decision in life, the right thing to do comes from what will feel amazing and true on the inside.

WHAT'S A-HEAD?

I think next week I'll do one of my final gray hair videos. I say "one of my finals" because I'm sure there will be other revelations that will come from this experience down the track and I'll want to share them. I also still have a final inch or two of dyed hair clinging to the ends so I'm not officially done. And last, given how my salt and pepper still seems to be a work in progress, it might be fun to take a long game approach and compare how it changes as time goes on.

In this "last" video I'll lean my head into the lens of my iPhone and let viewers look at my wires. Those pesky antennas seem to have given in a bit to gravity - *Ha, I showed them!* They've given up the fight as they've grown longer, relaxing rather than aiming for outer space. Then I'll play beauty vlogger for a bit and share that tip I mentioned before about only using conditioner to wash my hair. It's been a good one that still seems to work.

I'll for sure mention that finally, now that the dye is mostly off and I've found a way to care for my hair that I've also learned to embrace my natural curls. I haven't been able to for years because they were fried and hidden behind frizz. The last thing I wanted to see up until very recently was my "natural hair." I think there's something big in that because how many times in life do we try to change ourselves to be something we're not? How many times do we hate on the shape of a body part that really is never going to change regardless of how many crunches or squats we do when we should be so grateful that it actually works? Being okay with my hair, just the way it is, without anything to change its shape, is kind of like coming home.

Blocking out the vlog script, I think from there I'll put on my coaching hat and try to make sense of how trying new things, even when they're as superficial as only using conditioner rather than shampoo, going on the gray hair adventure in itself, can act like a gateway for questioning everything that we do on autopilot. I'll explain what that meant for me and how during this time I've experimented with life changes like getting more involved in what I eat and drink, what I put on my body and what I spend my time doing. Little changes that have added up and I think, at least I *hope*, have made me a better person. Like most of my videos, I'll throw down a challenge to viewers to maybe think about their own gray hair adventure, using it as a metaphor for questioning all the things they do out of habit. Maybe there's another and better way.

My gray hair videos have always gotten more views than the other vlogs that I put out each week on just about every "over 40's" topic under the sun. And even when one of those other videos gets watched - for instance the other day I did a video on coping with death - there's often a comment about how my hair looks rather than keeping with the subject. I got a couple of those on that one. I have to kind of smile. We're visual people and maybe we have to start with what we can see, what's on the surface before we're ready to take a breath and look at the foundation of all that stuff.

Or maybe I should've been a beauty vlogger. #toolatenow

I sometimes wonder what would've happened if my hair sprouted white rather than salt and pepper. Maybe that would've put a whole other spin on my thoughts and my experience. Perhaps that I got a gentle transition made me have to dig a bit deeper to the meanings behind this change. That digging deep became almost like a meditation for me, constantly thinking about concepts like kindness, aging, boundaries, esteem, vulnerability, patience and even enjoying uncertainty.

Granted, some of those lessons I've had to learn again and again and the jury is still out on whether I've become a good student. For example, I seem to still suck when it comes to learning how to communicate with hairdressers. A few months ago, I took a chance with getting my hair trimmed at one of the few local salons left that I hadn't blacklisted. I'd gone in there for a couple of blow dries in the past, the girl that worked with me knew I was purposely letting my hair grow out. I went in with pictures on my iPad of a trendy messy bob that should've been fine with my hair.

But the hairdresser got spooked, either by my curls or my age or that she really didn't get the gray hair thing I was after (that came out in our conversation which in itself should've had me cancel the cut) because rather than listening to what I wanted, she gave me a boring straight, safe looking "mom" cut. The hairstyle equivalent of "mom" jeans.

She could tell my mood had flattened as she blowed my hair straight. I couldn't smile. This whole hair thing is sometimes so bloody exasperating and exhausting! Perhaps some of it was the realization that even with a cut there was still a lot of dyed bits left. It was just taking so damn long!

But more than that, I was pissed at myself that after all these many months of talking about boundaries and dealing with authority figures like hairdressers, it was clear that I still couldn't stand my ground and get what I wanted, over the simplest, silliest thing.

Of course I made a video about it. But it was hard for me to do. Rather than banging it out in one take, I had to record it over a couple days because I was so dejected by how ridiculously hard it was for me to get what I wanted in, of all places, a beauty salon.

The good, and slightly crazy, news is that I took matters into my own hands once my hair grew out of the "mom" stage and I trimmed it myself. Oh yes I did. I just couldn't bare to go to a hairdresser again. I needed a break. I bought a pair of hairdresser scissors, watched a bunch of YouTube videos and went for it. It was thrilling. I felt like I beat the system. Truth be told, it wasn't the most perfect cut in the whole wide world, and for that hairdressers do have my respect for the magic that they can create, but it bought me a little time to think about how I'm going to get what I want the next time I do put my head in the hands of someone else.

Which reminds me of another beauty tip!

I've since learned that if you want your hairstylist to give you a cut that is NOT age appropriate, you definitely should let them know that you want to look "modern, young and fresh." That way, they're not going to make a judgment call on what they think will work for you and to be fair, this hairdresser always saw me as someone who was harried, going gray and busy. On my end I thought I was just busy. She seemed to want to give me something that was easy for me to put up in a rubber band and hide with. And to that I say: #missionaccomplished

Modern. Young. Fresh. I'll try that next time. And there will be a next time and a next time and a million next times after that. I won't give up on trying to have a successful, exciting, equal partnership with a good stylist. One who I can go to again and again. Maybe if I can do my part and learn how to *finally* speak the lingo, I'll get closer.

Oh, and then there's this.

Since I started this strange dye-free trip two years ago, there've been some changes in my hood. In the early days, it seemed entirely possible that real life "Cindys" were a figment of my imagination. No one was doing the gray hair thing. But the other day I was taking a walk and saw a striking model type, about my vintage, strutting into a cafe like a rockstar, her grays well overtaking her colored blonde. Five minutes later a gray haired badass ran past me, training hard and in the zone. And not long after that I crossed paths with a silver locked mermaid, drying herself off after a swim in the winter sea.

The timing of it all was pretty uncanny. I'm choosing to believe that seeing all these rapid fire visions of fierce women owning their attitudes, not to mention their natural hair color, was no coincidence. And in that moment I realized that through these two years, I got a backstage pass to understand how transformation happens. Slowly. One person at a time. One change of mind and attitude at a time. And then it's everywhere you look.

Winding up an adventure always makes me feel kind of humbled. After all the climbing and just dealing with whatever you need to do to reach the next point, you get to the summit. You get to finally throw off your backpack and take a look at the view and look at that long path that started as a tiny dot, full of questions.

Through this adventure I touched some unknowns. I learned about fear that I didn't know was there and I learned that being afraid is often about the monsters you create in your head. I had first hand experiences in where I felt like I had a good grip on how things evolved and others where there was *and is* definitely room for improvement. I came face to face with myself.

I think I get who I am as a person going into the second half of my life and it feels good, thanks to the most innocent of all things, hair color.

I think I also get who we are as a society in a time when a lot of the old rules about what's possible are falling away, thank goodness, all because of - you got it - hair color.

I know that soon, there will be something else that comes up. Something that pushes my buttons and asks me to put the backpack back on. But for now, just for this moment, me and my salt and pepper, steel gray in certain lights, but ultimately 100% naturally colored hair, will just sit down and take in the view.

Lesson Learned

Life is short. Have an adventure.

That is all.

The Gray Hair Adventure Videos

Here's a list and descriptions of the vlogs I made of my Gray Hair Adventure. You can watch all of them, and any additional ones that come out after this book, on my website at http://www.thechangeguru.net/grayhairadventure

#1 Let The Grays Begin

This was my first video in the adventure and I was fired up! I had just been to the French hairdresser who told me my hair was gonna look like "sheeeeet" if I stopped dyeing. I didn't intend to do regular videos about the journey but he certainly gave me the inspiration I needed to start it off. A little behind the scenes info, at the start of the video I include a Skype call I was having with my friend Lorane Gordon, a happiness coach. She didn't get why I would do such a crazy thing like ditching dye and she still doesn't get it, but she loves me anyway. A little side note, if I could've done this video all over again I would've done a few things differently with the main thing being, I wouldn't have gone for so long. I think I could've said what I needed to say in half the time.

#2 Sh*t People Say When You Grow Gray Hair

This video was done at about the three month mark. It's also the first one where I start wearing a silly hat at the beginning of the video so I could do a bit of a reveal of the current state of my hair. At this point my ears were pricked for all the things that people were saying about going the gray route. From my younger girlfriends (who are covering their own gray) to my own mother (who's still loving the dye), the comments say a lot about where we're at in our collective thinking and are a reminder that if we want to be perceived in a different way, we're going to have to speak up.

#3 Self Acceptance While Growing Out Gray Hair

This video was done at month five and the reality of what I was doing was starting to sink in. At the time I described the results of what it looked like this way," My gray hair is like a new born chook - it's coming in slowly, slowly. In some light you can see it big time, in other light I just look like a gal that has let myself go in the hair dye department!" This was the time where insecurities started to make themselves known. I had to act as my own personal coach to help me give myself the gentleness and compassion required for taking on something that is a physical adjustment.

#4 Gray Hair - Coping With Opinions of Others

This video was done during month six of ditching dye and I was just starting to come to terms that my hair was sproutin' wires! I described it this way," Seriously, it's not THAT drastic but I'm starting to move into the squirmy stages of how to manage hair that needs to learn how to behave. It's like having kids all over again!"

#5 Makin' Like Clooney When You Grow Gray Hair

Around month six, I started going after the often quoted
thought process that men look better with gray than women do,
that it looks "distinguished" and "handsome". It got me
thinking about what would happen if we actually co-opted these
descriptions, often used for men, as our own. Plus, I wear a
"moose" hat, a gift from my husband after doing a job at
Yellowstone National Park.

#6 Rock Your Gray Roots When You're Out On The Town

This video was inspired by noticing that my cousin's wedding
was coming up and it was going to be one of those times where
I'd be revealing my new "project" to the family I hadn't seen for
a while. In the vlog I offer up three mindset tips for taking the
emphasis off your hair and into the heart of the event.

#7 What If Growing My Hair Out Gray Makes Me Look Old?

Recorded at the nine month mark, this video was made after I saw some pictures of myself with my emerging hair. I looked older. Sometimes that's a moment that really gets to some people. For me it was a little out of body but I chalked that reaction and what I could do with it up to a learning experience. How I coped with these pictures was a turning point for how I now consider myself if I ever look "old".

#8 Gray Hair: Dealing With Wobbly Moments

Around month ten, the novelty of what I was doing had worn off. I was really on the path. This two-toned hair was a part of me and that was when I started getting scared. This was around the time when I woke up in the middle of the night and had to do a 3:00am reality check of all the good things in my life so I could get some balance to the scary thoughts that were racing through my head. I'll say it right here, like I say in the video and like I said in the chapter in this book, wobbly moments pass.

When in doubt, get a blow dry.

#9 Exploring Color When You Grow Gray Hair

Probably around the time I made this video, at month 11, I started to rethink some of the habits I'd locked myself into, especially with my looks. For years I'd worn a "uniform" of black everything. Black dresses. Black yoga clothes. Black bathing suits. My closet was full of black. And I felt tired of that. Tired of being so predictable to myself. I demonstrate an experiment using a color palette app designed to help you discover the best hues for your skin tone, eye and hair color. I figured now that my hair was no longer a majority of orange, less harsh colors than my basic black might be my new friends. While I'm not running around in a lot of strong colors I haven't bought anything black for a long time. Another example of how the gray hair adventure pushes you out of your comfort zone.

#10 Gray Hair: Activate Your Inner Badass

The concept of this video really summed up the possibility of ditching dye and growing your hair out gray. This was made at the 12 month mark, so it literally took me a year to fully own this feeling and it's stuck with me ever since. The concept of using gray hair as a badass statement seemed to really resonate with the women who watched it. We've been pushed with so much gray hair fear that permission to feel like a badass about it was huge. The hat I'm wearing was a present that Dale got me while he was working in Moscow and if you weren't sure, the word I say at the beginning of the video, is "Badass" in Russian. At least I thought it was at the time. I've since tried to find the translator that I used to get it and nothing comes even close. I maybe should've said "задира" which is pronounced "Zadira". So far, no one's corrected me so I'm hoping it's the gist that counts.

#11 Under 40 and Growing Gray Hair? What You Need To Know

After a year of connecting with women on the gray hair journey, I was given an education on younger women who were dyeing their hair, from a very early age. Like I was inspired by the Clooney's of the world, I also found that it was young women who were ending up being my style gurus. This video, made a bit over a year of not dyeing was my message to them.

#12 Things My Ex-Hairdresser Taught Me About Growing My Hair Out Gray

This one was made after my reunion with my French hairdresser. I remember at the time I was feeling so good and normal with my hair - which was great! - but creatively I was a bit blank when it came to what to talk about in my next update. Be careful what you wish for. Ha! The encounter gave me exactly what I needed and leads to a reminder for you creatives out there. if you ever get stuck, do something different. Go out and connect with someone. Have your coffee at a different cafe. See a movie in a theater rather than on Netflix. Chances are something will happen or be heard or be seen that will unlock whatever's kept you stuck.

#13 What If Your Gray Hair Doesn't Look Good Enough

This was the video where I sang my hillbilly version of "Am I Not Pretty Enough", a really sweet country song by the Australian singer Kacey Chambers. I use my umbrella as a guitar and reference Cindy Joseph in it. What a potpourri of crazy! The realization that my hair wasn't going to be the colors I'd hoped for was hitting me here and I used that comparison to all the other ways we don't feel like we measure up.

#14 Gray Hair: What You Need To Know About Haircuts

Poor me! This video was done in two parts over two different days. The first part I recorded just before I went in for that boring mom cut I described in the book. I was so happy before

I went in. Now, when I watch, I yell at the screen, "Don't cut it..." My intention was to video the new look as soon as I got back home but I was so bummed out that I couldn't give myself enough positive energy to talk. I needed to process it. So instead, I took that expensive cut and blow-dry and went straight into the ocean. I did the second part on another day after I was able to regroup. I was still feeling it and almost scrapped that take in order to wait a couple more days to try again. Keeping it real won the coin toss.

#15 Trying New Things When You Grow Gray Hair

I got the Mickey Mouse hat I'm wearing in this video from a recent plane flight that was doing a Disneyland promotion. Besides the fact that a Mickey Mouse hat is seriously one of my favorite kind of hats in the whole wide world, I was especially stoked to get those mouse ears, because I was completely out of hat options for any future videos. That's the first thing I thought of when I got it. *I love how the gray hair adventure is never far from my mind!* This video is special to me because I recorded it so close to the time I finished this book. I certainly never knew when I did my first video a couple years ago that I'd end up writing a book about the experience. A reminder that life is full of surprises, kind of an off shoot theme of the video topic itself.

Resources

My Favorite Gray Resources

Going Gray Looking Great Book :

http://goinggraylookinggreat.com

Cafe Gray: http://w11.zetaboards.com/Cafe_Gray/index/

BOOM by Cindy Joseph: http://www.boombycindyjoseph.com

Lauren Stein's Blog "How Bourgeois ":

http://howbourgeois.blogspot.com.au

Going Gray Looking Great Facebook Page:

https://www.facebook.com/Going-Gray-Looking-Great-

334857020776/timeline/

Revolution Gray Blog: http://goinggrayblog.com

The Way I Wash My Hair

Curly Girl Method (Co-Poo):

https://www.youtube.com/watch?v=NDofglvTFx8

Articles Mentioned

Katie Holmes Hair Has Flecks Of Gray article, Daily Mail -

http://www.dailymail.co.uk/tvshowbiz/article-2591016/Katie-

Holmes-35-reveals-flecks-grey-gets-tresses-transformed-ratty-

mess-voluminous-set-TV-pilot-Dangerous-Liaisons.html-

Women Sabotaging Each Other, Forbes -

http://www.forbes.com/sites/work-in-

progress/2011/11/30/the-psychological-warfare-of-women-

are-we-our-own-worst-enemy-2/2/

Dunning Kruger Effect - "Unskilled and Unaware of It: How

Difficulties in Recognizing One's Own Incompetence Lead to

Inflated Self-Assessments". *Journal of Personality and Social*

Psychology 77 (6): 1121–34

Thank you

First off I'd like to thank all the great women in The Change Guru community who've been there for me during my experience and have also shared their own adventures. I'm so glad that the gray hair adventure has brought us together.

Thank you to Diana Jewell, Cindy Joseph and Lauren Stein. These three women inspired me to take on this journey through their breakthrough work on the subject, long before I turned it into a project for myself.

Last but not least, all my love and gratitude to my family. You are everything to me.

WOULD YOU LIKE TO KNOW MORE?

If you'd like to know more about my Gray Hair Adventure,
come over to my website at
www.thechangeguru.net/grayhairadventure. You'll get heaps of
pics of my transition, all my videos, blogs, podcasts and links to
the resources I found most helpful for experience.

The best thing about connecting through my Gray Hair
Adventure is that it's one of the many unique ways I help
women navigate change after 40 whether it's life purpose,
wellness, relationships, career or family I've got heaps of
resources to help you thrive. To find out first on what I'm up
to, sign up for my newsletter list. Subscribers get freebies,
discounts and inside info.

Visit http://www.thechangeguru.net to get in.

DID YOU LIKE THE GRAY HAIR ADVENTURE?

Before you go I want to offer a personal thank you for buying my book.

There are a gazillion and twenty books out there and that you spent time with mine is huge to me. So heaps of gratitude for getting all the way to this point.

Now, I've got a little favor to ask that can really help me. Can you please take a quick moment to leave a review for this book on Amazon? Even a short sentence or two will make a difference. Your review will help inform other readers and gives me feedback to take on board for the future books I write.

Thank you!

More Books By Susan Paget

Be Your Own Change Guru: The Ultimate Women's Guide For

Thriving At Midlife

http://www.amazon.com/Be-Your-Own-Change-Guru-

ebook/dp/B00HU14CEM

How To Find Your Purpose After 40: The Secret To Unlocking

Your Unique Gift To The World

http://www.amazon.com/How-Find-Your-Purpose-After-

ebook/dp/B00LBMYU7A/

ABOUT SUSAN PAGET

Susan Paget is an author, online commentator and coach whose work focuses on issues that are important and life affirming to women over 40. A dual American/Australian citizen, Susan is the mother of three adult children and lives with her husband Dale and cat Cleo in Sydney, Australia.

email: susan@thechangeguru.net

website: www.thechangeguru.net

YouTube: www.youtube.com/susanpagettv

Facebook www.facebook.com/thechangeguru.net

Printed in Great Britain
by Amazon